18048

The Medical Student's Survival Guide 1

KT-416-493

The Library, Education Centre
Royal Surrey County Hospital
Egerton Road, Guildford, GU2 7XX
Tel: 01483 464137

Class number   W 18

Computer number H0806087

The Medical Student's Survival Guide 1
THE EARLY YEARS

ELIZABETH COTTRELL
Foundation Year 1 Doctor
University Hospital of North Staffordshire

Radcliffe Publishing
Oxford • New York

Radcliffe Publishing Ltd
18 Marcham Road
Abingdon
Oxon OX14 1AA
United Kingdom

www.radcliffe-oxford.com
Electronic catalogue and worldwide online ordering facility.

© 2007 Elizabeth Cottrell

All rights reserved. No part of this publication may be reproduced, stored in a retrieval system or transmitted, in any form or by any means, electronic, mechanical, photocopying, recording or otherwise without the prior permission of the copyright owner.

Elizabeth Cottrell has asserted her rights under the Copyright, Designs and Patents Act, 1998, to be identified as Author of this Work.

Neither the publisher nor the authors accept liability for any injury or damage arising from this publication.

British Library Cataloguing in Publication Data
A catalogue record for this book is available from the British Library.

ISBN-13 978 1 84619 086 5

Typeset by Egan Reid, Auckland, New Zealand
Printed and bound by TJI Digital, Padstow, Cornwall, UK

Contents

About the author

Elizabeth Cottrell, a Foundation Year 1 doctor, achieved MBChB (honours) while at medical school. Elizabeth learnt a lot from co-writing her first book, *The Medical Student Career Handbook*, during her final year at medical school. This invaluable experience helped her to develop the *Survival Guide* with national medical student involvement from the start. Elizabeth has drawn from her experiences, and those of other medical students to answer the questions of prospective and current medical students.

About the contributors

A few individuals deserve a special thank you for the vast amount of time, effort, work and support they have provided during the development of this *Survival Guide*. Each individual provided his or her time and expertise for nothing. The following individuals have been significantly involved in contributing to and critiquing chapters:

Dr Robert ('Bob') Clarke, Associate Dean for London Postgraduate Medical Education and 'a legend' to many medical students nationally. Also, thank you so much for your fantastic revision courses that helped me to become a doctor.
Ms Kate Frascr, The University of Manchester Medical School
Dr Basma Hassan, Foundation Year 2 in the West Midlands Deanery
Ms Pauline Law, University of Dundee Medical School
Mr David Little, The University of Manchester Medical School
Mr Vishnu Madhok, University of Dundee Medical School
Dr Christele Rebora, Foundation Year 1 in the London Deanery
Mr Imran Sajid, The University of Manchester Medical School
Ms Laura Stevens, University of Dundee Medical School
Mr Paul White, University of St Andrews Medical School

The following individuals contributed to the content of the *Survival Guide*: Allie Blair (The University of Liverpool), Rachel Boyce (University of Aberdeen), Nat Bradbrook (The University of Manchester), Zoe Cowan (The University of Leicester), Stephen Domek (University of East Anglia), David Douglas (University of Dundee), Esther Downham (University of Dundee), Kate Geraghty (The University of Leicester), Anna Kieslich (University of Dundee), Elizabeth Li (The University of Manchester), Jemima Miller (University College London), Oliver Shapter (University of Aberdeen), Ross Stewart (University of Dundee), Katie Thorne (The Hull York Medical School) and Alexandra Williams (University of Leeds).

Acknowledgements

Thank you to Dr Charlene Kennedy, Foundation Year 1, who encouraged me right at the start, when the *Survival Guide* was just a bubble of inspiration floating around my brain!

Ms Sharon McConville provided a wealth of information and advice about eating disorders and medical students. This is an important topic and the work of individuals like Sharon is much under-recognised.

A thank you must also go to all my peers, colleagues and patients who have provided me with the material, inspiration and experiences from which the book is written.

Finally, a thank you must go to my husband, my friend and my rock, Paul. Without his support, help and encouragement I would not be the happy wife, doctor, daughter and sister I am now.

CHAPTER 1

Introduction

> Medicine is a vocation in which a doctor's knowledge, clinical skills and judgement are put in the service of protecting and restoring human well-being. This purpose is realised through a partnership between patient and doctor, one based on mutual respect, individual responsibility, and appropriate accountability.
>
> In that day-to-day practice, doctors are committed to:
> - Integrity
> - Compassion
> - Altruism
> - Continuous improvement
> - Excellence
> - Working in partnership with members of the wider healthcare team.
>
> These values, which underpin the science and practice of medicine, form the basis for a moral contract between the medical profession and society. Each party has a duty to work to strengthen the system of healthcare on which our collective human dignity depends.[1]

Medical school is fantastic, fun and fulfilling, but it is also tough. It may mean leaving home, fending for yourself for the first time and it is mentally and physically challenging.

The welfare subcommittee of the British Medical Association Medical Students Committee (BMA MSC) carries out regular surveys on national samples of medical students to assess medical students' welfare. The results of the 2006 Medical Students Welfare Study[2] will be referenced throughout this *Survival Guide*. Although the survey is not bias-free, important information can be gleaned from it, such as some hazards of being a medical student. Being aware of such hazards will help you to avoid them, for example:

➡ medical degree study having a negative effect on personal health and well-being
➡ using alcohol to cope with pressures of work
➡ stress negatively affecting health.

To succeed at medical school, you need to work harder than you ever imagined. Your role and your presence will not always be appreciated and you will have to mature quicker than many of your non-medical student peers. That said, medical school offers unique, intriguing and humbling experiences and opportunities. Few other degrees offer such insight to the lives of other people; this will make you very worldly wise. Medicine provides the buzz of success, the heartbreak of tragedies and mental and ethical challenges that go hand in hand with caring for, diagnosing, treating and managing patients and their friends and relatives.

Two medical student survival guides have been developed to provide you with realistic insights into undergraduate training. *The Medical Student's Survival Guide 1: the early years* contains information on the 'pre-clinical' years at university. *The Medical Student's Survival Guide 2: going clinical* is targeted at medical students entering the later years of their course, the majority of which will be delivered in a clinical setting. Although it is recognised that this split is not clearly defined in many medical schools, information contained in each *Survival Guide* is signposted in both books to assist you to access the relevant information. The content has been informed by the enthusiasm, experiences, challenges and successes of the author and UK medical students. The *Survival Guide* may not always provide solutions, but confirmation that your views, experiences and problems are not unique. Medicine and medical training is constantly changing and evolving. Therefore use the information within the *Survival Guide* to help you to be proactive in finding up-to-the-minute information.

The *Survival Guide* will not guarantee you a pass in your exams; however, it will provide you with information that will make the day-to-day experience of being a medical student much easier.

Each *Survival Guide* contains quotes, thought bubbles, speech bubbles, arrows and stars.

➡ Quotes by UK medical students and literature: opinions, thoughts and advice that demonstrate the diversity of experiences and advice that occur throughout medical training.
➡ Thought bubbles: examples of questions you should ask yourself.
➡ Speech bubbles: questions commonly asked by tutors/examiners or useful phrases to try out when appropriate.
➡ Arrows: action to take to further your experience, knowledge or practice.
➡ Stars: important, key knowledge for undergraduate students to grasp during medical school. Not exhaustive, but signpost important concepts and illustrate the level of understanding required of you.

Appendix I contains *Resources*, a directory containing comprehensive contact details for relevant organisations. Contact these organisations for detailed and accurate information.

Standards addressing admission to medical school, finance, education, support and careers were laid out by the Medical Students Committee (MSC) of the British

Medical Association (BMA), in *Medicine in the 21st Century: standards for the delivery of undergraduate medical education*.[3] These standards highlight the expectations the MSC have of medical schools and students (now and in the future). The Council of Heads of Medical Schools (CHMS) and the BMA have set out further standards (Appendices II–V) that medical schools and medical students should strive to meet.[4] Familiarity with these standards will ensure you meet expectations and receive all you are entitled to.

> When applying to medical school many potential students declare a 'commitment to lifelong learning' to demonstrate their desire to obtain a ticket to the marvellous journey that medicine provides. But what are the different routes, diversions and delays that today's medical students face, and are these causes for concern?
>
> Medical students have to build a commendable CV in an environment where competitiveness and ambition is rife; passing written and clinical finals is simply not enough to join the bottom of the medical career ladder. So what can a medical student do to distinguish themselves from the plethora of cloned colleagues? Get work published? Intercalate? Join their Medical School Committee? Evidently competitiveness is an aspect of any career pathway, although there must surely be a feeling of déjà vu with personal statement writing and UCAS applications in the not-so-distant past for final-year students.
>
> Another concern inherent among students is that of finances. Medical students are unusual as it is normal to spend up to six years completing an undergraduate degree. Demanding clinical timetables and gruelling revision regimens leave little scope for medical students to take on part-time employment. With several banks now offering professional loans of up to £20,000 and interest-free overdrafts the opportunity for medical students to accumulate dangerously high degrees of debt often receives attention from the media.
>
> We must remember that the vocation of medicine is not a one-way ticket, and there are indeed many routes that may be taken before reaching the desired destination. Many doctors will reminisce about their turbulent journey and several places that they otherwise would never have had the opportunity to see while stopping en route. However, what remains evident is that 'commitment' must be a prerequisite before boarding. (*Vishnu Madhok, fourth-year medical student, Dundee*)

FURTHER READING

MacDonald R. Rhona's rules (on what being a medical student and doctor is all about). *StudentBMJ*. 2004; **12**: 458–9.

CHAPTER 2

Medical school: the early days

STARTING AT UNIVERSITY
Maps

> Campus maps are essential pieces of kit. No point turning up for a lecture in the wrong building! (*Pauline Law, first-year graduate medical student, Dundee*)

Unless you have chosen to go to university in a familiar area, one of your first purchases should be a local street map. Campus maps are provided to all university students and highlight the buildings you will be attending for university-based teaching, most university-based social events but usually not clinical placements. You may receive campus maps as part of a Fresher's pack, during an open day or application process or they can usually be accessed on the internet. You may have to visit a family home early in your first term and you will run the risk of getting lost or being late if you do not have a good street map. In addition, you will need to buy food and perform other activities of daily living: without a map you may know the street of your favourite supermarket but not know how to get there.

> Don't do what I did in my first week and turn up at the nearby HILTON hotel instead of the Hilton Building for a lecture! (*Vishnu Madhok, fourth-year medical student, Dundee*)

If you are going to be relying on public transport, try and get hold of a transport map. These are often available from bus stations, train stations or tourist information centres. Using public transport is easy if you have a rough idea of how to get there and where it is. Do not forget, when travelling by bus you can always ask the driver to call out your stop when you reach it.

Respect for your new surroundings
Consider the locals

It is not just students who live in the area of your university. Local residents may resent students when facilities become crowded and the area becomes more noisy and disrupted. Making sure you behave well and respecting the local population is even more important as a medical student as you will be relying on your local residents for your education (they are the patients). It will be hard for a local resident to consent to you taking their blood if the night before they saw you unconscious on the pavement in a drunken stupor or in a fight.

As a medical student it will be rewarding and enlightening to obtain an understanding of the local population and the area's history. You will often be surprised and amazed at the stories residents tell of their lives. The history of an area has a great impact on the health of the residents at the present time; for example, students studying at Keele University medical school in Staffordshire will see many 'dust-related' lung pathologies in the old pottery workers and coal miners. Indeed, ignorance to the previous existence of coalmines in the area would result in Keele students being unable to explain "mining tattoos": small, permanent, black marks just under the skin caused by miners rubbing against the coal face.

Safety and crime

Respect for your surroundings does not just relate to doing no harm. Become safety aware and 'streetwise' when you go to university. Universities are often in cities. If you are used to living in a quiet village, where you can leave your house unlocked and use your mobile phone while getting cash out of a machine, then you need to learn how to keep safe and do it fast.

One in three students becomes a victim of crime while at university.[1] Over one in ten university students living in private accommodation experiences a break-in.[1] Bicycles are a common target for thieves as are mobile phones and, increasingly, personal MP3 players.

Below are some tips on keeping safe and to try and prevent yourself becoming a victim of crime while at university.

➡ Do not use your mobile phone in the street unless absolutely essential. Muggers will punch victims in the face while taking a mobile phone that is in use.

➡ Never use cash machines alone.

➡ Be wary of strangers approaching you, especially if they are asking for money (e.g. for telephone box or bus fare) or if they have just seen you leave a cash machine.

➡ Lock everything. This means your accommodation *every* time you leave it, your car and/or bicycle. If you are living in halls, it is a good idea to lock your bedroom door when you leave it (even to go and get a meal for yourself). If your house has a double lock or alarm use it, or both.

➡ Do not come home alone from a night out. If you are living in halls this is usually easy, you will usually live in the same place as at least a couple of people you are out with. If you have to come home alone, pre-book a taxi.

➡ Empty your room of valuables during holidays. Whether you are living in rented accommodation or halls, take valuable items back home with you or put them in secure storage (often available in halls).

➡ Carry a personal alarm. These are easy to obtain, drug-company representatives sometimes give out free ones and some universities provide them free of charge.

➡ Be careful who you let into your accommodation. If you are staying in halls with security doors, do not let other people in with you unless you know them or have seen their identification.

Register with a GP

You are responsible for maintaining your own health (*see* Chapter 14); as a medical student it is a fitness to practice requirement. In addition, university residences and universities like you to be registered with a GP and have this information on file in case you become ill. Find and register with a GP as soon as possible after you arrive at university.

You will be able to find GPs in your local area on the websites www.nhs.uk/ England/Doctors/Default.aspx, www.show.scot.nhs.uk, www.wales.nhs.uk and www.healthandcareni.co.uk. Find somewhere that is local to your accommodation, so you do not have to travel far when you are sick. Health centres are available in universities, and you may be able to register there if you are living on-campus.

Photos for ID purposes

Identification photographs – these will be with you for five years! And they will be sent to everywhere you go on placement and are put up on the walls in hospitals and medical schools, on ID cards and so on. The numbers of people who sent in photos they have regretted ever since (school photos, looking spaced-out, dodgy pictures that look like police photos). A good photo will save you years of embarrassment! (*Stephen Domek, third-year medical student, University of East Anglia*)

There are many reasons for which you will require photographs over your first few weeks at university. Your medical school and the societies and clubs you join request them, mainly for identification purposes and club cards. During the first term keep a few passport-sized photographs with you at all times to avoid long waits at university photo booths.

Friends

Friends are the most essential piece of kit for surviving medical school. In the first few weeks say 'Hello' to everyone, accept every offer for a get-together that you can – the first few weeks are the time when people try themselves out in groups. Not everyone you have a coffee with will become a bosom buddy, but when you are about to enter a dissection room for the first time it is easier if you know that deep down everyone else feels the same. A network of colleagues to get together and bounce ideas around, or share useful websites with, or even just 'Oh my God, I don't understand that' will make the dark days seem brighter. (*Pauline Law, first-year graduate medical student, Dundee*)

Many people at university are away from home. Many have not gone to university with their friends. Therefore, many people have the potential to be lonely. You are all in the same boat so take advantage of this. Be open and friendly with all. Acquaint yourself with a number of people. A good opening to any conversation is asking where they are staying – you may even find people with whom you can travel to and from university and social events.

Do not expect to make best friends in the first few weeks. In fact, many of the people you may speak to during the first month may fade into the myriad of faces belonging to 'the people at university you recognise'. However, through people with whom you do not 'click' you may meet others with whom you do. With so many medical students, let alone university students, you are bound to find a really close friend. Just remember these things take time – do not despair.

MISSING WHAT YOU HAVE LEFT BEHIND

Never forget those you have left behind – during holiday times, those people who've burnt their bridges will be the ones watching Bank Holiday television when you're out with your friends – home friends can be useful to you whilst at university, too. It's good to have someone to talk to who isn't there, who's removed from the situation. You can moan about the gruelling medical course and, in return, you can listen to the moans they have about their life. I often find my home friends give the best advice. This is particularly good if they aren't at university at all, but are working or still at school. (*Laura Stevens, first-year medical student, Dundee*)

Many medical students have moved away from their home town or city. Some may be relishing the thought of leaving parents behind, making new friends and discovering new surroundings, shops, clubs and bars. Others may be a little more apprehensive.

You cannot predict the people who will have difficulty coming to terms with moving away. Even those who appear easy going, confident and friendly at school may struggle to find their feet. Past confidence may be a result of the total acceptance that comes with long-term friends, thus having to make new friends can be daunting.

I remember keeping a radio on in my room for the first few weeks to break the silence. *(Vishnu Madhok, fourth-year medical student, Dundee)*

Students who have moved to the UK to study from foreign countries may be at the greatest risk of loneliness and homesickness. Great distances make home visits difficult; the result being an even greater desire to go home. Overseas students also have to learn about a new town or city, country, culture and, in some cases, a new language. This makes even normal activities difficult.

The moment you are first on your own and away from home is very memorable. It is a feeling of excitement, nervousness and anticipation, balanced with varying strengths of 'what have I done'. Overwhelming loneliness may lead you to be on the phone all the time, have your radio on constantly or watch more TV than is good for you. However, these feelings will often soon pass as you meet other people in the same situation, discover people you already know are at your university and become so busy that you have little time to look back.

You are most likely to feel lonely, homesick or both when you need the support of people who know you. This may be the first night, when you feel uncertain of making new friends, or it may be around exam time. Whenever it happens it will be unpleasant and upsetting. However, given time you are likely to build supports with the new people you have met at university.

Although you will be caught up in a whirlwind of nights out, excitement and new experiences, you will regret it if you lose contact with those people who know you best. It can be difficult to adjust to friends from home moving on. They will be living life, doing the things you used to do together, with other people. But you have to remember you are not in their lives either any more and they are going to be missing you just as much. Your home friends may even miss you more as they are used to having you around. Everything you are experiencing is new and you have never done it with your home friends. You need to learn to use the time you have together well, and keep in touch so you do not miss out on the news from back home.

If things get really difficult and you are incredibly lonely or homesick it can affect your academic performance as well as making you totally unhappy. Therefore, do not be ashamed, worried or shy about seeking help and advice. All universities have personal welfare and health services; you could also talk to a tutor you trust at the medical school, a mentor or your own GP (*see* Chapter 14).

CADAVERS

Dissection – a tricky business! Choose the weeks you volunteer to get your hands dirty carefully. Cracking the ribs and sternum with tools more suited to your local mechanic can be fun, but delving into the unknown mass of the gluteal region – a hidden cave of wonders that can splurt the less agile with a face full of dead juice or produce copious amounts of fat if your subject's girth happens to be on the wider side – is definitely less appealing. On the other hand, jigsawing the cranium at full pelt just to have your anatomy demonstrator yell out (only to the ears of the audience as you are deafened by the power tool) that you should stand well back as the brain (plus all attached gooey bits) makes a mockery of your lab coat does have a certain charm. *(Elizabeth Li, second-year medical student, Manchester)*

Dissection is a famous component of medical school education. How many times have you told someone you are a medical student only to be met with the response 'Do you cut up dead people?' However, not all medical schools include dissection in the curriculum. In 2006, two medical schools had to drop dissection from the curriculum because of a lack of body donors.[2] Therefore, if you have strong feelings about the inclusion of dissection during your time at medical school you will have to investigate whether the schools you are interested in will have it on the curriculum while you are studying there.

Dissection is a wonderful learning opportunity should you be offered it. Before you have been into an operating theatre, dissection will be the first time you witness what lies deep within the body. You will marvel at the colours, greens, yellows, pinks and purples, and you will be astonished at the size of organs – both larger and smaller than your textbook-informed mind had you imagine. You will never feel the need to learn the normal weight and dimensions of an organ, when you have seen it you will never forget it. Problem-based learning (PBL) courses are increasingly common; however, students who have undertaken their studies via PBL courses are perceived to have poor anatomy knowledge.[3] True or not, you should really make an effort to grasp the opportunity for taught anatomy with both hands. Dissection is the perfect platform for this.

We spent four hours per week in the dissecting room in semester one, and this commenced in week one, so it was important that we could discuss our feelings – a lot of students were really apprehensive about the dissecting room and were worried that no one else was at all concerned about it. *(Laura Stephens, first-year medical student, Dundee)*

So how will you cope when you face a dissection room for the first time? Not sure? No one is. Nothing can prepare you for the first time you enter a room full of dead, preserved bodies. However, most people, bar a couple of minor hiccups (or should that be faints), usually cope very well. The anticipation is worse than the reality and once you get going with the lesson you no longer think about the 'dead people' but the fascinating sights.

If you do feel ill in a dissection class, tell someone straight away. It is better to admit it and sit down than faint and land headfirst on the corner of the dissection table or in the dissection specimen!

The worst thing for most people is the smell of the room. The bodies are drained of blood which is replaced with preservative. This has a distinctive smell that many people find unpleasant. For some it is not a problem. Just wait and see.

Your involvement in the dissection will depend upon you, your tutor and the organ/system being studied. Generally, you can volunteer to cut or extract the required parts of the body. If you are happy to watch at first this is acceptable, just make sure you can see everything that is going on. Occasionally your tutor may perform some of the dissection if it is particularly delicate or intricate, so you do not cut through the structure you are looking for and ruin the usefulness of the specimen.

If you have recently been bereaved or, for some other reason, you think dissection will be too painful to participate in, let your tutors know. You can discuss your feeling with your tutors who will have experienced such situations before and will be able to help you if things get difficult.

> You could sense the nervousness, an army of first-year students in matching lab coats, as they trooped into the dissection room for the first time. The smell of anticipation, nearly as potent as the formaldehyde, both lingering in the air and on everybody's clothes long after they'd left the room. Unspoken questions filled people's heads: What will the cadavers look like? Do they smell? Is mine going to be male or female? Some students, unperturbed by the experience, were eager to get going. Others, like me, had their reservations. However, by the end of two hours I'd nearly forgotten that the tissue I was cutting and pulling once belonged to a living, breathing member of society.
>
> Two weeks on and the dissection room does not scare me quite as much. However, I still haven't forgotten that the cadaver was once a man with a history, a family, a life. I will never know his past or even his name. Still, I can't help but wonder. It really has made me consider the concept of life and death. At what point did this man become a body? The moment his heart stopped? The moment he was declared dead? When his family said goodbye? When he was preserved? The line is not clear-cut.
>
> What would he think of us, the group of first-year students, armed with scalpels and only a rudimentary knowledge of the human body? Is he looking down on us, shaking his head when we accidentally cut through a nerve we should have preserved? The life after death argument is complex, and at the end of the day our views on this are unimportant. Regardless of what we think, we are privileged to be able to study the body, a gift given by someone who wanted to make a difference.

I hope that the families of the cadavers in the dissecting room are grieving with feelings of admiration for their family member. By donating their bodies to medical science, those people have given a huge gift to us. Who knows, some of these students may become world-class surgeons or pioneering researchers. I think if those people are looking down on us in the dissecting room, they'd be proud. (*Laura Stevens, first-year medical student, Dundee*)

FRESHERS WEEK

Talk to as many new people as possible; you never know which of them will become your friends in the future, or who you will end up working with. (*Laura Stevens, first-year medical student, Dundee*)

Freshers week, occurring in the week before the true university year, is the highlight of many students' undergraduate years. Although aimed at newcomers, many senior students return to university a week early to participate in Freshers activities. Although it is stereotypically about drinking, Freshers week is actually designed to help settle new students into their new environment.

Drinking!

Getting drunk seems to be synonymous with Freshers week for many students. To say 'do not drink' is silly; however, if you do drink do it safely. Think about the recommended drinking limits for men and women and be aware of how much you are drinking (*see* Table 2.1).

TABLE 2.1 Information for safe drinking[4]

Recommended safe drinking levels depend on personal factors, such as health and body weight:	
Men	21 units per week
Women	14 units per week
Definition of binge drinking:	
Men	5 or more drinks on one occasion
Women	4 or more drinks on one occasion
Units* (vary between different manufacturers, strengths and are reliant on precise measures):	
Pint of beer	2
Pint of cider	2
Pub measure (25 ml) of spirit	1
Pub measure (50 ml) of sherry, port	1
Alcopop	1.5

*One unit = 8 g or 10 ml of alcohol.

If you are drinking do not get separated from your friends. You may only be newly acquainted, but you should look out for each other. Take the phone numbers of the people you are with so you can contact them if you do get split up. Similarly, do not leave a venue on your own. You are very vulnerable and suggestible when drunk. Taxis are not only cheaper but also safer when you share them.

Look after your drinks. Do not leave drinks unattended and try to get bottled drinks so you can put your thumb over the top while you are holding it. You can now buy special tops to insert into the neck of a bottle that makes securing the opening easier.

Only you know your limits when you are drinking. However, it is a good rule of thumb that if you have had a few drinks and then suddenly decide it is a good idea to have a few more or 'do shots' your body is really telling you to stop. There is no fun in ending your night with your head down the toilet.

> Think about the type of people you want to be with, what clubs and interests do you have? What is going to look great on the CV in five years' time – and is it something you enjoy? Then make the time to get there.
> (*Pauline Law, first-year graduate medical student, Dundee*)

Joining clubs, societies and organisations

Although there will be societies you will want to join for fun, there are also some medicine-related societies that may interest you. Joining medicine-related societies is often cheaper (or free) as a student than when you are a doctor so take advantage of this so you know which memberships you want to continue when you have to pay full price. Some societies (mentioned below) have great student offers and added extras that are only available to members. Below are a few societies/organisations you may wish to join.

British Medical Association

The British Medical Association (BMA) is the professional association for all UK doctors with sole negotiating rights for doctors. It represents doctors from all branches of medicine all over the UK. Student members receive a monthly copy of *StudentBMJ*, containing interesting political, lifestyle and educational articles, and opinions of medical students accompanied by *Student BMA News*, featuring news, views and analysis. For full details on the benefits of membership, visit the BMA website (www.bma.org.uk/join).

> Do everything you can, and early! Join societies, volunteer for local charities, play sport and do not neglect the hobbies you had before medical school. You will meet people from all walks of life and be thankful for some 'non-medic' conversations when your life increasingly revolves around hospitals. It will also help with job applications; cramming in new

hobbies in your last year to boost your CV could be really stressful. (*Kate Fraser, fourth-year medical student, Manchester*)

Medical Defence Union

The Medical Defence Union (MDU) is a mutual, non-profit organisation that provides members with advice and support throughout their studies and professional lives. Benefits of membership include access to a Freefone 24-hour Advisory Helpline, discounted books, courses and educational services, and access to case histories and advisory publications within the MDU website. For further information about the benefits of MDU membership visit the website (www.the-mdu.com).

Medical Protection Society

The Medical Protection Society (MPS) provides its members with medico-legal advice and assistance, and protects them in an increasingly litigious climate. For student members, the Society has developed a scheme that provides support while they are training. This includes discounted medical textbooks and free educational materials, worldwide elective protection and editions of *Casebook*, the MPS members' journal full of risk management ideas, case scenarios and news. You can also access revision courses for your final year examinations through the MPS. Visit the MPS website (www.medicalprotection.org).

Medical and Dental Defence Union of Scotland

The Medical and Dental Defence Union of Scotland (MDDUS) is a professional indemnity organisation that has been protecting the interests of doctors and dentists since its foundation in 1902. Although based in Scotland, the Union looks after members throughout the UK. The role of a medical defence organisation such as the MDDUS is to provide you with medico-legal support and advice in the event of a claim of medical negligence or a complaint being brought against you. It is a legal requirement that you have professional indemnity in place before starting out in your career. When you graduate you will face a number of unfamiliar situations and there may be times when you feel you need some advice or reassurance. During your university years, you may also find yourself in unfamiliar situations. Student members of the MDDUS have full access to clinically qualified medical advisers 24 hours a day, 365 days a year. Student membership for the MDDUS is free. The student membership scheme was set up to introduce students to the benefits and services of the MDDUS at the start of their university life. Through this, student members receive a free MDDUS diary, discounted books from clinical textbook publishers, a free MDDUS quarterly newsletter, sponsored educational and social events throughout your university years and free worldwide indemnity cover for overseas electives. Visit the website (www.mddus.com).

It is worth bearing in mind that should you encounter problems with your fitness to practice during your time at medical school the BMA, MDU, MPS and MDDUS may be an invaluable source of advice and support.

Freebies

Freebies are a massive benefit of Freshers week. Granted, you have to wade through lots of leaflets, free passes to terrible nightclubs and approach many stalls, but it is worth it. Walking round with your matching plastic bags, you and the rest of the university population will feel part of a club whose members will be spotted a mile off. Being a medical student gives you access to an even more exclusive club, as you will get fantastic free gifts from medical organisations and societies. This can include anything from a pen torch, personal alarm and desk lamp to free textbooks.

Generally, you can expect money-off vouchers and free food and drink. If you are smart (and sneaky) enough you will be able to get through the first week spending very little on nights out and buying hardly any meals (providing you do not mind drinking cheap vodka and eating instant noodles with free pasta sauce!).

Poster sales

Poster sales are a common occurrence within student union buildings and are invariably present during Freshers week. Here you will find hundreds of cheap posters; whatever your taste there will be something there for you. Poster sales are excellent places to go to help decorate a dingy student house or a stark university hall room. However, make sure you know the rules of your accommodation regarding sticking posters on walls or you may be liable for a fine when you leave.

The student union nightclub

Wherever you go to university, your student union nightclub is likely to be popular, cheap and contain people just like you (and their friends!). However, descriptions of many student union nightclubs often include the words *dirty*, *sweaty*, *tacky*, *grimy* and *meat market*. Student union nightclubs can make a fantastic night out, they may provide transport to university accommodation, host great themed nights and are usually full, due to the cheap drinks and good advertising among the student population. Wait and make your own judgement when you go, but do not expect it to be a classy night out!

The Ball

Freshers week often culminates in the Freshers Ball. These vary in formality between medical schools: some may be black tie events, others may be more casual. They are usually huge events. Expect one of the best nights of the year. Famous or tribute bands often provide the music and fairground rides may be there to entertain you. Let your hair down, have fun with your new friends and make the most of it, this often marks the beginning of the hard work!

STUDY

⫸   **Proper Preparation Prevents Poor Performance**

> Medical students should be aware that they have to start working from the start. I say this with hindsight, as my exams are next week and I am totally unprepared, having not worked enough earlier in the semester. Keeping up-to-date with reading and work throughout the term would have made the exam period a whole lot easier. (*Laura Stevens, first-year medical student, Dundee*)

Work starts early in medical school. Not only this, but you will be studying a subject that uses an entirely different language for a large proportion of time. While most university students on other courses have a prolonged Freshers period – of up to three years in some cases! – medical students often find themselves on full timetables within the first two weeks of term. Make sure you are always near to a medical dictionary in the first few months and learn the meanings of all new words as they arise; otherwise, you will soon fall behind.

> If you have been away from studying for a while the sheer volume to cram in is intense. Starting to learn/revise basic anatomy and physiology before coming to medical school or in the early days would have been a great idea. Some people sat a pre-med year, but I didn't have time for that. (*Pauline Law, first-year graduate medical student, Dundee*)

As with all university courses, the medicine degree course is designed with the expectation that you will be self-motivated. Kickstart this motivation during the early days of medical school otherwise it will become very easy to slip into a 'student lifestyle' of drinking as soon as you finish university and getting up late to watch afternoon television with your breakfast. If you do this at the beginning you will miss the basic concepts that you need to learn in order to have something on which to build your future knowledge; this time will not be regained easily. Perhaps those most at risk of falling into unhelpful 'student' routines may be those coming from backgrounds of strict parenting and who relish the freedom university provides. Although you should not miss out on student living, be aware of turning 'dossing' into a habit.

An additional problem with study in the early days comes for those who may have taken a gap year or are mature students. It can be difficult to ease back into a routine that includes a huge amount of studying, especially if you have become used to stopping at the end of the working day.

Equipment

Depending on the nature of your course you may need various pieces of medical equipment. Medical schools often organise stethoscope sales at the beginning of your clinical years; however, there may be other pieces of equipment you need or think would be useful. There are a number of websites (for example www.medisave. co.uk) that sell medical-related equipment. If you are in a well-established medical school, you may find local shops that sell medical equipment. Items that you may find useful during your course include:

➡ stethoscope
➡ pen-torch – you can often get these free from drug company representatives
➡ white coat – for laboratory work and for clinical work
➡ ophthalmoscope (instrument used to examine the back of the eye) and otoscope (instrument used to examine the ear) – these are relatively expensive and usually not mandatory pieces of equipment; however, they are commonly examined techniques that you may want to get practise in.

FURTHER READING

Smith R. Thoughts for new medical students at a new medical school. *BMJ*. 2003; **327**: 1430–3.

CHAPTER 3

People you will meet

Although stereotypical and not exhaustive, this chapter introduces some of the people who will feature strongly in your medical training and career. It is recognised and appreciated that you will be spending time with various other professionals not covered here. It is also recognised that respect for all is the only way forward.

MEDICAL STUDENTS

Medical students come in various shapes and sizes. Many cannot be set aside from the people you meet away from medical school, however you may notice some of the groups listed below.

Quiet studious types

The quiet studious medical students are always calm, pleasant and appear content. They never seem flustered, stressed or arrogant. They study quietly and know much more than their modesty allows them to let on. They usually pass and do well but do not always get the top marks. An admirable quality of the quiet studious types is their diligent attendance at many of the medical student socials. You will never see them drunk but they will be present throughout the night.

> **Tip:** these medical students are often forgotten or ignored, but are some of the most well-rounded, pleasant people at medical school. Make the effort to get to know them and you will find a good source of decent conversation.

Noisy studious types

The studious students who tell everyone about what they know are, perhaps, the most unhelpful acquaintances you will have at medical school. Around exam time these students list everything they know, how well their tutors have told them they will do and talk about the minutiae of (what seems like) every condition. They boast about everything, even if it does not qualify a mention. Although they do well at their studies and achieve high grades they let everyone know about it. These students are easy to spot by listening out for someone loudly telling everybody about a time when they treated a patient single-handed and diagnosed a condition no one else had even considered.

>   **Tip:** ignore their boasting and displays of knowledge; they are only mentioning things they are confident about, just think about all those things they are not mentioning (I promise you, these omissions will be multiple).

Ravers

Ravers appear to do very little work, go out every night and try to persuade everyone to do the same. No one else can understand where they get their time, energy, knowledge or money from. Such medical students pass their exams with sickening frequency. This way of life is not recommended.

>   **Tip:** let them get on with it, do not feel pressured and be firm if they start bullying you to go out when you really do not want to or cannot afford it.

Those for whom a medical degree is a mere formality

There are some medical students who believe the minute they don their white coats and stethoscopes (only to remove them as soon as they realise it contravenes the image they are trying to put across) believe they are doctors. They think they know it all, deserve respect and can instruct the nurses on the ward. This is a bad attitude that will get them nowhere.

>   **Tip:** these medical students will trip up, upset the nurses and be put back in place by consultants; distance yourself from them in the clinical situation, especially if they regularly overstep the line.

The ladies' man

There are only ever one or two per year. For the ladies' man, becoming a medical student and doctor is desired to further enhance their already slick image. They will drive around in expensive cars, which even their parents cannot afford, trying to charm *all* the female student doctors and nurses – and getting nowhere with most of them. However, their 'charm' and chat-up lines will usually be a good source of amusement so we cannot knock them. You will spot them easily – to all females a confident 'hello' will always be accompanied by a wink.

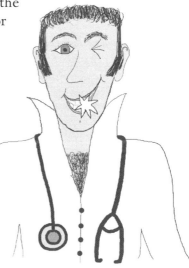

>   **Tip:** watch and laugh, it *is* funny.

Those who just get on with it

There is usually a small group of students in every year who form strong alliances with each other. They are not interested in the status or power of being a doctor, they do not get involved with the game-playing and they pass their exams comfortably. They know how to balance work and life, without spending all their life with people from work and/or in the pub.

Tip: students in this group are usually true to themselves, find someone you like and it will be a sincere friendship.

General medical student traits

One quality develops in all medical students. 'Bad handwriting' you all cry out. No: hypochondria. It is very difficult for the fertile minds of medical students to read about the weird, wonderful and worrisome illnesses that afflict the human race without considering the possibility that they are suffering from each. A spot becomes a cyst or an abscess, perhaps even the start of meningococcal septicaemia. Stomach ache becomes appendicitis and, if suffering with pins and needles, the poor medical student briefly contemplates a future suffering from multiple sclerosis. However, medical students often also suffer from pride. They know that it is ludicrous to think that they have leukaemia if they notice a few bruises that cannot be explained, so the anxiety remains unspoken. Treat medical students suffering ailments with care. Someday you may be in the same position as them and who knows what you will think you have got?

Romantic lives of medical students

Just as you would find in any large group of people, thrust together through good and hard times, romances start to develop. Do any of the following sound familiar?

Long-term relationship

High status medics (e.g. ravers or popular students) get together, work together, join societies together and live together. These relationships last, at least through medical school. Both people remain popular among their friendship group but do not make any effort with other medical students.

Playing the field

Female medical students who play the field tend to go for the blokes associated with the athletics union, rugby and hockey teams. They quickly establish this status by showing the males how much they can drink, attending all athletic union events and asking a different male to 'walk them home' at the end of each night. They thus have a good source of drinks throughout medical school.

Male medical students tend to play on the student DOCTOR part of their status.

They use this, and their potential 'fortune', to attempt to attract young nursing or physiotherapy students. They attend every medical student social with a different mute blond on their arm.

Ongoing inappropriate encounters

Ongoing inappropriate encounters usually involve medics with boyfriends or girlfriends not at university or who are at university elsewhere. These medical students are loyal and caring about the said boyfriend or girlfriend until they are on a medics' night out. After half an alcopop, these students gravitate to each other ('we are safe, nothing will happen, we are both taken') and soon end up becoming inappropriately involved with each other. They develop great levels of regret later in the night and the next morning, which lasts until the next medical social.

Why all this is important

> As a medical student you are forced to sit (in close proximity) with a group of medical students, some of whom you may not like (for a variety of reasons); yet you cannot leave the group or go off and work alone. Sometimes there is no way to improve the group dynamic. I have tried and so have some of my group members, yet it remains antagonistic and hostile – this is what I have to look forward to every day of my training. (*Anonymous*)

Medical school can be tough. Some of the toughest experiences result directly from other medical students. They are a competitive bunch and some have harsh and underhand traits. If you are finding 'being with medical students' difficult, read the above. Try and spot the different groups among your peers and have a giggle. You will see that you are not alone in having problems.

CONSULTANTS

> ⫸   **Consultants are getting younger, or am I just getting older?**

Consultants, like all the groups of professionals mentioned, are varied. They have different degrees of scariness, attitudes to medical students and are susceptible to having bad days. Few 'nasty' consultants now exist. You are rarely going to be humiliated on a daily basis. However, some do have nasty tempers, and you should try and stay on the right side of these.

> Just remember, like that merciless Doberman down the road from your childhood, consultants can smell fear. (*David Douglas, fourth-year medical student, Dundee*)

Old-school consultants will not understand, nor appreciate, your 'new-fangled course'. If you are undertaking problem-based learning (PBL) be prepared for comments about your lack of knowledge on basic sciences and your 'touchy feely' teaching. Consultants can generally be classified on the basis of their being surgeons or medics.

> The traditional surgeon was often caricatured as a man of the flesh – bold and beefy, handy with the knife and saw – little better than a butcher and no more learned than the barber with whose trade he frequently doubled.[1]

Surgeons

Surgeons require arrogance to be able to do their job. This is not a flippant comment. It takes a degree of arrogance to enter an operating theatre and cut open a patient. However, *displays* of arrogance are not essential; this accounts for the variation in surgeons from those who are unassuming to those who display arrogance in the cringeworthy, peacock-tail-like way that many medical students have to be accustomed to. Other common features of surgeons are: being male (although this may soon change), having flash cars and the ability to sing, out of tune, through an entire three-vessel coronary artery bypass operation.

Surgeons are often uncomfortable alone. They like to collect as many hospital staff as possible before they join a patient at their bedside. By the time all the followers have collected neatly around the bed, found a space and are ready to hear some pearls of wisdom, the surgeon will turn quickly on his or her heels, having finished their consultation, and leaving a flurry of paper, unwritten notes and flustered junior doctors in their wake.

Medics

> A superior physician plumed himself as being marked out by mind not muscle, brains not brawn.[1]

Medical physicians are usually very thoughtful, calm and methodical. They have an art of diagnosis and healing that involves doing, seemingly, very little. They have few followers on ward rounds (as few people have the stamina) on which each patient's case is considered carefully and each problem is addressed. Medics are the masters of history and examination and much can be learned of these skills from them.

Teaching style

Teaching styles may vary greatly. To perform well you must quickly discover your current consultant's preferred method.

Bedside teaching. Your examination and abnormality detection skills will be put to the test as you practise examinations of patients with good or discrete signs. Some consultants will let you complete the examination before asking you questions and evaluating your performance. Others will interrupt you all the way through. Find ways to cope with the latter to prevent it from becoming annoying and confusing, causing you to forget what you are doing.

Sit-down teaching method. In a room away from patients you will discuss a particular topic or get a mini-lecture. They may talk you through the topic step-by-step by asking questions.

Other teaching styles and focus of teaching depend upon the clinical setting, such as in theatre (basic anatomy), clinics (investigation, interpretation and management plans) and on ward rounds (holistic assessment of the patient).

Whatever your consultant's primary teaching style, make sure you are well prepared and enthusiastic. If you know you are going to be covering a certain topic or examination, study and/or practise it prior to the teaching session. If you are attending a ward round, make sure you know some patients well enough to present them if asked. Before going to theatre, take the time to look at all the patients' X-rays and scans, when appropriate, and study the applicable anatomy. It is not unheard of for a doctor to ask a medical student to leave a clinic or theatre if they are not adequately prepared.

GENERAL PRACTITIONERS

General practitioners are usually a nice bunch. Often more quiet and unassuming compared to the harshly competitive hospital doctors. GPs get a rough deal among medical students as they are commonly criticised by hospital consultants. However, you can usually get very good teaching from a GP as they know their patients so well. A good GP is invaluable to patients and thus will be highly respected and well appreciated as a result.

NURSES

Many nurses are knowledgeable, professional and excellent members of the healthcare profession. However, there are exceptions and, as a medical student, if you do not spot them they can either make your life a misery or you will be missing out on some good social-life potential.

Femedicophobes

Femedicophobes are always female nurses and are lovely ladies, but only to nurses, physiotherapists, social workers, bed managers, male medical students, male doctors . . . in fact, anyone who is not a female medical student or doctor. No matter what you do, you will not be able to win a smile.

Tip: stay clear if you are female, you will not get anywhere with them (except more annoyed) no matter how hard you try.

Older nurses

Older nurses have often worked on the ward so long they are practically running it. They usually have a wicked sense of humour and do not like jumped-up medical students or doctors.

Tip: in order to have a laugh with them, and not be the butt of their jokes, be good, pleasant, hard working and offer to make cups of tea.

Younger nurses

Fun, eager to learn and good for making friends to go out with or just to find out where the good places to go out are. Help each other to learn together if you hit a problem.

Tip: be yourself – friendly and approachable, it is a win–win situation.

Specialist nurses

Specialist nurses can be a fantastic resource to medical students. They often know their patients better than anyone else, they know their stuff and you can help each other along through difficulties or problems as you both have a different knowledge base. However, they are not doctors so do not always appreciate the responsibility of doctors or have the same training base as doctors. This can result in conflict and negativity in both directions.

Tip: appreciate, rather than resent, these individuals, you will gain much more.

BED MANAGERS

Bed managers are sometimes viewed as bulldogs with clipboards. However, this is unfair; they, too, are working to targets, primarily getting the new, sick patients into beds. Because of their demands for quick discharges aimed at busy doctors once the patient is fit to go they can be a source of irritation; but they are only doing their job.

Tip: bed managers are not doctors, nor should they dictate when patients leave. Allow them to inform you or your team that beds are required but do not allow them to bully for a patient's discharge before they are ready.

PHYSIOTHERAPISTS

Physiotherapists are often sporty-looking individuals. Their anatomy knowledge is usually far superior to the average medical student, and they will be the delightful people who will get even unmotivated patients up and about as soon as humanly possible. Without physiotherapists patients would be rendered immobile after a long period of bedrest, blood clots would be growing throughout all the legs on the wards and chesty coughs would be allowed to fester without being addressed.

Tip: physiotherapists are your friends with whom you can learn and work together to get your patients in tip-top condition.

PHARMACISTS

Pharmacists are perhaps the most pedantic members of the healthcare staff. They walk round with an endless supply of green ink, with which they scrawl countless corrections, notes and instructions across each and every drug chart you ever encounter. However, they have an important job, they spot many a prescribing mistake made by doctors and can be life-savers in this regard. Learn from the instructions they write and use them as a good source of pharmacological knowledge.

Tip: do not let their perfection gall you to the extent that you hate them for being so right.

DRUG REPS

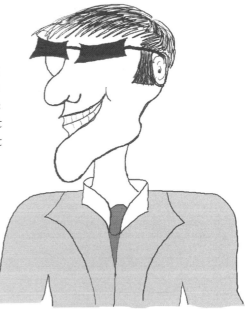

You will recognise the drug rep very easily – usually a pair of legs sticking out from under a huge pile of food. On the rare occasions that drug reps are attending a place of healthcare without food, you will recognise them as the most energetic, happy and suave people in the vicinity. Dressed impeccably and apparently interested in everything about you, you will be in no doubt when a drug rep is about.

The role of drug reps is to educate doctors and other healthcare professionals on the actions, benefits and uses of their company's drugs. However, their more famous role is to provide money, food (quantity and quality are both usually unnecessarily high) and free gifts for virtually anything. They crop up everywhere from GP's surgeries to hospital-based multidisciplinary team meetings. Controversial, but famous, are drug rep dinners, during which you 'endure' a short talk on certain products before sitting down to a (free) three-course meal.

It is up to you and your conscience to decide how much you take advantage of the 'free gifts'. There is much debate on how ethical it is to eat from drug rep buffets, take 100 free Post-It notes or 500 free pens. These freebies have to be paid for by something, and it is the NHS that picks up the bill by paying for the drugs the companies are promoting.

If you do partake in drug-rep freebies, please do so with restraint. It is not a pleasant sight to watch a medical student fighting with two nurses and a professor over the last chocolate doughnut. Similarly, it is not really necessary to have 15 desk lamps or three stethoscopes.

UNIVERSITY STAFF

Most university staff do not know (and often do not care) that you are training hard to be a doctor. You are just another student who is going to mess up the place, want things and make a noise. Be it a lecturer, secretary, library or canteen staff, you may be viewed with some distaste. You will soon learn which staff you can rely on to be rude and unhelpful.

> **Tip:** be nice to these staff regardless of how they treat you: you are certain to get complaints if you are rude to them; they quite literally know where you live!

FURTHER READING

Dean E. Received a gift? It's time to perk up. *BMA News*. 2007; **March 10**; 7 [outlines the rules about pharmaceutical company gifts and hospitality].

Prescription Medicines Code of Practice Authority: www.abpi.org.uk/links/assoc/pmcpa.asp

Salvage J, Smith R. Doctors and nurses: doing it differently. *StudentBMJ*. 2000; **8**: 176–7.

Thomas JD. Medical students: a spotter's guide. *StudentBMJ*. 2002; **10**: 340–1.

CHAPTER 4

Competitiveness

Competitiveness is a predictable feature of life at medical school. How does it manifest? How can you cope with it?

> Competition has been a driving force in the evolution of mankind. Competition is not necessarily beneficial in the short term; indeed, it can make our lives exceedingly difficult. It can cause us to compete for the sake of competing.[1]

DEMONSTRATION OF COMPETITIVENESS

All medical students have an element of competitiveness; this drives their motivation to work harder than others. However, competitiveness may be directed in two ways, internally or externally. Internally directed competitiveness is that which manifests as students wanting to do well for their own satisfaction. Students with externally directed competitiveness try to demonstrate that they are better than their peers through direct comparison or by trying to make other students look bad.

IS COMPETITIVENESS BENEFICIAL?

> The instinct for competition plays a role in every branch of human endeavour . . . natural talent is rarely enough for the true geniuses and high achievers in any field. Talent is often accompanied by persistence, a willingness to take risks and a burning desire to be the best.[1]

Medical students commonly work in pairs or small groups. Such high levels of talent and enthusiasm must breed intelligent discussion, sharing of experiences and increased knowledge due to mutual co-operation. Is this the reality? No. So why do medical students let competitiveness prosper over joint education?

The hypothesis outlined below works on the basis that medical students commonly work in pairs and that medical school exams often do not have a set pass mark but pass/fail thresholds that are derived from the exam scores obtained by the cohort of students (e.g. a pass may be the mean mark and a distinction may be the score which lies two standard deviations from the mean). Therefore, a fixed proportion of students will always fail and medical students are directly competing against each other. In this situation you are most likely to get the highest grade if your score is significantly better than everyone else's. In a highly acclaimed book, *The Selfish Gene*, Dawkins[2] describes a gambling game called the 'prisoner's dilemma'. It is on this concept that this hypothesis is drawn.

The two options medical students have are: (1) to share (knowledge, information or details of interesting cases, etc.) or (2) not to share. It is rarely obvious which medical students do each, as you will never know what the other is holding back. You cannot therefore work on a solely tit-for-tat basis. The medical students each have two options resulting in four possible ways in which a pair of medical students can work together.

1   Student 1 and Student 2 share knowledge, information or details of interesting cases.
2   Student 1 and Student 2 do not share knowledge, information or details of interesting cases.
3   Student 1 shares and Student 2 does not.
4   Student 2 shares and Student 1 does not.

Option 1, two-way sharing, results in maximum educational benefit for both students. Each makes sure the other discovered the rare and unusual patients, each gets equal practice of clinical skills and each would help the other if they were struggling. What is the drawback of this option? Both students may end up being equal and achieving similar scores in an exam. This would result in neither particularly standing out from the other. Standing out is important to competitive individuals and also in future job applications.

In Option 2, neither student has co-operated. Neither benefit from this as opportunities will be missed, topics will not be learnt and both students may have wasted much time playing games in order to make sure accidental sharing of information did not occur. Not only is one student stopping the other from learning, they are imposing a detrimental effect on their own learning as their own uncertainties will not be addressed. Neither student will do as well as they would have done if they had been working individually on the attachment.

Option 3 and Option 4 are the same, in essence, so will be discussed together. In this situation one medical student is willing to share and co-operate and the other is not. This is most beneficial to the student not sharing as they will reap the benefits of their peer's work and they will not be passing on valuable knowledge. Therefore, the student not sharing may gain much higher exam results than the (kind, giving) sharing student. This situation is likely to occur as a result of a conscious decision of a very competitive medical student. There are clear gains to the non-sharing student. In addition, the actual decision to share information is commonly not a conscious one. Medical students who try to work with their peers, rather than constantly competing against them, often cannot help themselves from speaking up when asked questions, asking their own questions or mentioning interesting cases or patients. These students also get pretty fed up of partners who do not share and quickly move on. Options 3 and 4 are thus often temporary arrangements, after a short while the partnership will split.

This hypothesis indicates the detrimental effects of competitiveness. Competitiveness may make students lose sight of what they are aiming for. You should not be at medical school to get the highest marks or to outwit other students but because you want to be a doctor. The most constructive use of competitiveness is striving to be the best doctor. To achieve this, concentrate on communication, empathy, good work–life balance, appropriate attitude and the multitude of other topics covered in this book.

To summarise, competitiveness may assist you to get good grades in exams or to stand out from your peers; however, it does not necessarily make you a good doctor. Think about which option you and your clinical partner fall into. Is your current behaviour beneficial for your exams, future career or patients?

> The reality of medicine is that medical students can be very competitive. Many do not like sharing information or answers to questions. This runs contrary to the whole ethos of medicine, of being altruistic and working in a group. Before I started my medical degree, I would have defined myself as 'a team player', someone that likes to help others. Now, I have learnt that I need to work alone and keep valuable information to myself as I am in competition with my group and classmates. (*Anonymous*)

WORKING AND COPING WITH COMPETITIVENESS
Low self-esteem
The effects of your peers' competitiveness will depend upon whether it is externally or internally directed. If your peers are constantly comparing themselves to you in a negative way, it can be damaging to your self-esteem. Try and stay away from these people, especially if you lack confidence.

Unhappiness
Low self-esteem can lead directly to unhappiness. Unhappiness may also arise from frustration about the lack of co-operation between your peers. You may have identified that life would be easier and more beneficial if you all worked together but you cannot make this happen. Talk to non-medical student friends. You need an objective view, opinion or shoulder to cry on when things get tough. Maintain non-competitive friendships and hold them with great value.

Inability to congratulate peers on achievements

Competitiveness leads to bitterness when others do better than you. Rather than just recognising how well your peers or colleagues have done, you feel you have failed, they do not deserve the success or they have cheated. This is a great shame – be happy for others when they do well as you would like them to be for you. Rather than being bitter, learn from your peers' achievements. What have they done? How have they done it? Could you do something similar? Accept the fact that sometimes you will do well and sometimes other people do. Their success does not reflect on you at all. If you want to be the best put the effort in. Do not put other people down to raise your profile. Your competitiveness can be more constructively channelled into motivation.

Game-playing

Games occur when students try to make their peers look bad in order to make themselves look better. For example, they may not pass on messages about teaching sessions, say the wrong time for ward rounds or clinics and leave difficult procedures for peers to do when they completed all the easy ones (thus increasing failure rates among peers). Do not get involved in game-playing and treat your peers as you would expect them to treat you. If you have information to share then share it. If you have found an interesting case or a useful piece of information, let your peers know. Lead by example if you have any hope at all of changing things. Do not expect miracles. You may feel used at times, as many medical students will take and never give, but you may just break the cycle of information-withholding with one or two other students.

Missed opportunities

Concealing information and game-playing will result in missed opportunities and thus will have a damaging effect on education. You need to keep your ear to the ground and be proactive to stop your peers damaging your education.

Dishonesty

When students want to look or do better than everyone else, an air of dishonesty can arise. Some people may state experience they do not have and others will make up lies about their peers as part of a game-playing process. Be true to yourself and others and take what other people are saying with a pinch of salt unless you know them well.

CHAPTER 5

Attitude and behaviour

A guide to a desirable attitude to work, life, colleagues, patients and everything!

> The old catchphrase that describes the two traditional phases of medical education . . . 'precynical' and 'cynical'.[1]

During medical school you should develop attitudes and behaviour that are suitable for a doctor, including those towards the general public, specifically, patients and colleagues.[2] In addition, the Council of Heads of Medical Schools (CHMS) and the British Medical Association Medical Students Committee (BMA MSC) remind students that they are in a 'privileged position with regards to patients and those close to them'. As a medical student, you are expected to maintain a good standard of behaviour and show great respect for others.[3]

Worryingly, attitudes of medical students (e.g. towards doctor–patient relationships and communication) consistently reduce during medical school.[4] This is a serious problem. Read, understand and follow required standards regarding attitudes and behaviour; *see* Appendix II and *Duties of a Doctor Registered with the General Medical Council*.[5] Review both sets of standards and reflect on the extent to which you conform to them. If changes are needed, take them seriously. Your attitude can damage future doctor–patient relationships, thus undermining your work as a doctor.

> The purpose of medicine is clear. It is to care for the sick always and to cure patients where possible; it is to prevent ill health and to treat disease; it is to promote well being and create healing environments. Professionalism lies at the heart of being a good doctor. It sets a standard for what patients should expect from their medical practitioners.[6]

PROFESSIONALISM

Professionalism is one of the most important skills you should master during your medical training. Recognised as such, the Royal College of Physicians (RCP) published *Doctors in Society*[6] to outline professionalism in the changing world of medicine. It is well-written, easy to read and will provide you with a foundation on which to base your attitudes and behaviour throughout the rest of your career. *Doctors in Society*[6] describes medical professionalism as including 'a set of values, behaviour, and relationships that underpin the trust the public has in doctors'.

Hilton and Slotnick[7] described six areas in which you should demonstrate professionalism:

1 An ethical practice. *Duties of a Doctor*[6] and *Good Medical Practice*[8] are good sources of reference for this. You can access these documents from the General Medical Council (GMC) website (www.gmc-uk.org).
2 Reflection and self-awareness. Reflect on your own practice. Be aware of how you act around others, colleagues, patients and peers. Improve weak areas.
3 Responsibility for actions. Never blame others for your actions.
4 Respect for patients. Patients deserve the respect and treatment that you would want. Regardless of their situation, they require non-judgemental, appropriate, useful and empathetic care.
5 Teamwork. Demonstrate teamwork within peer groups and wider, multi-disciplinary teams. Learn how to lead and be part of a team. Respect the roles and importance of each team member.
6 Social responsibility. Understand your social responsibilities, as well as those of other team members and the healthcare system within which you work.

Acquisition of professional behaviour involves observation of other professionals, active learning of what is expected of you, education in medicine itself and reflection on your behaviour.[6] Be aware of negative role models and insufficient support which lead to unprofessional behaviour.[6] Reflection encourages awareness. If you notice your own negative behaviour, or others have expressed a concern, seek help and advice from an appropriate tutor/senior immediately.

Medical students who exhibit unprofessional behaviour at medical school are more likely to undergo disciplinary proceedings during their future career.[9] Medical schools use assessments and feedback forms to gain an impression of your professionalism from those you are placed with. Learning professionalism will thus benefit you now and in the future.

WORK

|||➡   **The best predictor of future behaviour is past behaviour.**

A desirable attitude to work and work–life balance is difficult but valuable. It is easy to forget that you are at university to learn how to be a doctor, not just to pass the exams. Work hard on the wards and undertake the everyday duties of a doctor while simultaneously studying comprehensively. Medicine should be part of, not your whole, life. It is acceptable to not want to 'do medicine' all your waking hours.

Your appropriate work–life balance will depend on your desired end goal. You may want to learn everything in great depth, in which case you may settle on a work-weighted work–life balance. If you are happy to 'just pass' your exams but also live much of your life away from medicine, then your work–life balance may be more equal; either is acceptable, providing you are clinically and professionally competent and you are happy with your life.

Take work seriously, no matter how well you want to do in the exams. Be encouraged to incorporate humour but meet all deadlines and attend compulsory sessions. No one is above these rules. Breaking the rules makes you look arrogant, unmotivated and uninterested.

It is hoped that medical students will be interested and enthusiastic about medicine but it is inevitable that you will not enjoy and be stimulated by everything. Please remember that sessions, clinical experiences and specialties are in your medical student curriculum for a reason. Try to attend all non-compulsory sessions when applicable to you. You are likely to learn something and it is rude to waste the tutor's time by not turning up.

> In the competitive world of medicine there is a strong tendency to try to be 'the best'. But simple mathematics shows that everybody cannot be the best: there is only one best . . . you should aim to be a good enough medical student and doctor.[10]

Interest will maximise your gains from any experience through making you receptive to information and encouraging your tutor, teacher or colleague to share information. If you are not enjoying the experience, politely engage as best you can.

All medical students must take psychosocial issues, seminars and lectures seriously. You may believe that psychosocial training is 'commonsense' or 'waffle'. However, when you get out into the real world, many psychosocial concepts help you to understand the behaviour, reactions and mood of some patients. Discussion of psychosocial components of a patient's history also really improves case reports.

Reflection enriches all experience. Do not accept situations or teaching without questioning why it is so; *see* Box 5.1. Reflection is not a useless buzzword, but an incredibly important tool that you should regularly use to regulate your work, life, attitudes, clinical abilities and career. Reflection may prevent you from being judgemental, ensures greater understanding of basic, general and medical knowledge, and increases the benefits gained from any experience. Reflection should be undertaken after any patient encounter, following negative/positive experiences, as part of a formal appraisal or assessment process and when making lifestyle or career decisions.

Box 5.1 Points to reflect on
- Why did that patient behave like that?/Why did this happen?
- How did you handle the situation?
- What did you do well?
- Could you have done it better?
- How would you do it next time?
- How did someone else handle the situation?
- Was it done well?
- What can you learn from it?
- What made you feel happy/relieved/unhappy/awkward/confused/angry today?
- Why did you enjoy/not enjoy the day?
- Can I see myself doing . . . in the future?
- If so/not, why?
- What would I do if I were in the patient's position?

Your placements and clinical activities may have accompanying assessments and/or activity sheets required by your university. It will only be you that looks bad if you do not complete them properly. Keep all sheets up to date. Fill them in throughout the placement to ensure accuracy. Be honest when completing clinical activity sheets, forms or a self-assessment of your competencies. If you have not been doing enough, reflect on your attitude to work and clinical placements rather than being dishonest. If you think ward experience is pointless and you can learn more from daytime television, remind yourself that the aim of your course is to become a doctor. It is possible to reach graduation having rarely attended a ward, but this will be of no use when you are responsible for the lives of others.

Honesty, probity, call it what you will, but remember to value it whatever you are doing. Honesty is encouraged in the medical workplace by the 'no blame culture'. Mistakes should be owned up to, apologised for and learned from. Without honesty systems cannot progress.

Cheating

There are many things that students can be forgiven for; dishonesty is not one of them. A zero tolerance of cheating among medical students is generally accepted. If you believe cheating is acceptable, think again. A pattern of dishonesty at medical school continues forward into work, with patients and colleagues, and with other regulatory and professional organisations. Medical school tutors understand this and will act quickly to eradicate dishonesty and those who practise it.[11] No one automatically deserves to be a doctor; the position should be earned with integrity.

Cheating includes:
➡ direct copying of others' answers during an exam
➡ taking notes or memory cues into exams
➡ talking about exams just undertaken to those about to take it
➡ obtaining non-official past papers
➡ plagiarism
➡ lying on application forms.

To avoid being unfairly accused of cheating:
➡ do not take mobile phones or any other communication device into exam rooms
➡ do not write anything on your hand on the day of an exam (even if it is just a reminder you need to buy milk on the way home)
➡ only use revision material that has been published nationally and/or released legitimately
➡ seek advice on referencing and using published texts in your work if you are unsure
➡ *be honest*.

PLAY

Student fitness to practice and medical student registration are relatively new concepts that may result in your life in and out of medical school being scrutinised. Medical schools (and the GMC) may become responsible for disciplining you for 'out of school' antics potentially affecting your future career. Be careful of your actions when you are out and about.

Criminal activity is unacceptable. Those with whom you have a drunken argument in town may be patients or visitors on your ward the next day. Act respectably, particularly if your placements are in a small community.

Aside from these warnings, do not take life too seriously. For some older doctors, failure to follow this is their biggest regret. Sometimes seriousness is a necessity at work but not at play. Take hold of non-medicine activities with both hands, relish a life outside a hospital or GP practice. These 'real life' experiences will enrich you with a greater confidence.[12]

PATIENTS

Without patients, doctors and medical students would be obsolete. Patients are the most important people in medicine. Your attitude towards patients should always be appropriate and constructive despite your (lack of) experience. Medical students should be aware that their contact with patients is usually for personal benefit not that of the patients.[3] Put yourself in the position of the patients: How would you feel? How would you want to be treated? Use these questions to shape your attitude.

Patients call the shots for everything comprising their care, including a medical student's involvement. Do not be offended when patients refuse your presence. On many occasions patients lay their emotional and physical self out on show, naked for all to scrutinise and ponder. Being witness to this is an amazing privilege; not a right. Conversely, you must learn a certain amount by the time you qualify; not only to pass your exams but also to be a competent and confident doctor. So do not encourage your patients to refuse you, which may be tempting if you are nervous or unsure of your capabilities.

Be aware of your patients' rights. Understand and practise informed consent and confidentiality (*see The Medical Student's Survival Guide 2: going clinical*). Appreciate and consider the ethical rights of patients, and thus the ethical responsibilities involved in patient care.

A common but undesirable attitude that can develop or be demonstrated is prejudice. Prejudice is a preconceived idea about a patient or group of patients that has arisen without reason or experience. Prejudices can arise as a result of, for example, a patient's lifestyle, culture, religion, political beliefs, ethnicity, gender, sexuality, disability, age or socio-economic status. Prejudice leads to negative behaviour such as discrimination against the target group or individual. Prejudice has great potential to affect patient care. It is thus crucial that you recognise your own prejudices; if we are truly honest, we all have some. Recognising our prejudices helps us to respect patients as we can stop these attitudes adversely affecting our behaviour.

Be open-minded. A lack of arrogance complements this quality very well. Who are you to judge how a patient came to be in their current situation? Your job is to understand. Make yourself aware of the diverse lifestyles within which people live.

You may not approve of all, but this is irrelevant. Open-mindedness overcomes prejudice, prevents discrimination and allows you to treat every patient equally.

Unfortunately, many medical students and doctors develop undesirable attitudes. Importantly, medical students have been shown to lack empathy for patients.[13] Privately they may ridicule a patient's situation, joke about their afflictions or remain flippant about emotional turmoil. So what causes people, who have entered a caring profession and know the importance of respect, to develop these attitudes? It seems that some negative attitudes may actually be part of a protective mechanism. Only rarely do young people in the developed world have to cope with the quantity of death and suffering that faces medical students. Indeed, bad things happen to good people. Undesirable attitudes towards patients may not be acceptable but are a manifestation of a distancing process that has to occur in some form to maintain a good, general mental health. If you realise that your attitude towards patients is changing in a negative way, find new ways of dealing with distress as a matter of urgency.

> You have to realise early on that you are no longer the best. Whereas in your A level classes you will have been within the top one or two students, now, you are not. You are in a room *full* of 'top one or two' students. (*Laura Stevens, first-year medical student, Dundee*)

PEERS

Attitudes of medical students towards their peers are sometimes shockingly negative. The following statements may be familiar to senior medical students:

⮕ **'Always be proactive in seeking out the best learning opportunities. This may mean being forceful to the point of saying "I'll go with doc X in this clinic" and then just going. Don't sacrifice your learning for somebody else. Realise it is a harsh world and that everyone else is doing the same thing.'**

⮕ **'Never tell any other student any fresh ideas you have for patient presentations. They will copy you. If you are assessed against your peers then make yourself as attractive as possible. Be an individual . . .'**

Uncooperative attitudes such as those exhibited above often stem from the continuous, underlying competition that is consistent within medical careers (*see* Chapter 4); competition for exam results, job applications and recognition. Students often want to work individually rather than working more effectively together. Such attitudes are self-perpetuating among the medical school population. If medical students are at the receiving end of such an attitude they may adopt it for themselves. Has this happened to you? Respect and treat others as you would want to be respected and treated yourself.

> Cliques and snobbery are not the way forward! *(Rachel Boyce, third-year medical student, Aberdeen)*

PROFESSIONAL COLLEAGUES

You will learn much of your clinical knowledge from colleagues and peers. Through appropriate interaction you can discuss, learn and problem-solve your way through most situations. To gain a broad and thorough knowledge base, interact with many different healthcare professionals.

Identify the professionals involved with your patients' care and introduce yourself. This will open a two-way communication channel. Recognise all healthcare professionals as the equals that they are. Effective patient care is reliant on co-operation between multi-disciplinary team members.

Integration with the team is the key for education. You do not, and never will, know it all. You will learn a lot from nursing staff and house officers. Many medical students adopt the stance that their role is not basic patient care, nor is it menial administrative tasks, therefore they do not participate in such activities. Do not forego educationally useful experiences to record blood results, but assist colleagues when nothing else is happening, especially if the ward is busy. You will gain more respect by helping than you would by standing around doing nothing and being in the way.

If you are an integrated team member, staff will approach you when they want bloods taken, ECGs recorded and cannulae inserted, thus providing you with the opportunity to practise your clinical skills. You will get first-hand information on patient management plans, including investigations required, procedures and tests; take these opportunities to assist, observe and experience new situations. Full integration with the team will increase the chance that patients view you as a useful part of the team and not just as someone who wants to use them as practise material. This removes many barriers you may otherwise face.

Valuing effective integration into the team with which you are placed removes barriers, results in a full understanding of the activities within your team, increases your confidence, consolidates your knowledge and ensures you know about any interesting events that occur, thus enriching your learning experience.

Recognise the usefulness of working closely alongside the junior doctors in your firm, which is excellent preparation for when you start work. Medical students can carry out many of the junior doctors' activities but have the safety net of being closely supported, something you may not have when you qualify. In addition, you will learn the tricks of how to carry your jobs out smoothly and efficiently, thus making life easier when you are in their shoes.

IRRATIONAL FEARS AND DISLIKES

Do you have any irrational fears and dislikes that you have encountered during medical school? Does it affect how you behave around certain patients or when encountering a particular problem. You need to develop your own way of overcoming these because, as a doctor, you can be faced with the good, the bad and the ugly at any time. Current medical students have laid themselves open to agreement or ridicule on their irrational fears and dislikes!

The good

⟱ 'Communication skill videos are never as bad as you think they are going to be!'

⟱ 'Everybody gets totally scared before giving an oral presentation, but everyone always does a good job. It is horrible while you are there but no one will notice you shaking!'

The bad

⟱ 'Cotton wool and cotton wool-based dressings never used to be a problem, but now . . . touching it, watching it being ripped or even cut just makes me squirm and/or wretch.'

⟱ 'I cannot believe it, I have just graduated and one of my peers still cannot stand the sight of blood – how have they managed?'

The ugly

⟱ 'I cannot stand veins . . . this may present a problem on a vascular ward!'

⟱ 'Toenails . . . I cannot stand them, especially old people's toenails when they have fungal infections . . . uugh!'

FURTHER READING

Persaud R. How to improve your motivation at work. *StudentBMJ*. 2004; **12**: 365.

CHAPTER 6

Course structure

> The core curriculum must set out the essential knowledge, skills and attitudes students must have by the time they graduate.[1]

This chapter explains the different aspects of medical courses; the general structure of medical courses and the 'extras' that can be added on to your medical degree. Each medical school is different; however, the general principles remain the same and these will be described. Each course curriculum contains a core component and a number of student-selected components (SSCs) (*see* Chapter 15).

The medical degree is vocational, that is, it leads you straight into the medical profession. It is designed to be intellectually challenging, to place increasing demands on you and to provide a foundation for your work as a doctor.[1] You are not expected to know everything when you leave medical school; however, you should know how to gain appropriate knowledge in the future.

> One of the great things about my course is the timetable. There are two semesters a year. In the first two and a half years it is half-day Monday to Friday. This leaves plenty of time for work, play and sleeping. To accompany a regular timetable there are additional clinical skills workshops and seminars. (*Zoe Cowan, first-year medical student, Leicester*)

KEY CURRICULUM GUIDANCE

Doctors are expected to work in accordance to the General Medical Council (GMC) *Good Medical Practice*[2] guidance. In relation to this, the GMC produced a document, *Tomorrow's Doctors*,[1] which sets out the curricular outcomes. It does not matter how these outcomes are met, but they must all be achieved in order for you to graduate. *Tomorrow's Doctors*[1] clearly states that the *Good Medical Practice*[2] guidance should be the basis of medical education. A medical degree will not be awarded to people found to contravene these guidelines in their undergraduate years. You are advised to read the full *Good Medical Practice*[2] guidelines; however, a summary of them may be found in Box 8.1 (*see* Chapter 8). *Tomorrow's Doctors*[1] explains the outcomes required of medical students that fall under each of the categories listed in Box 6.1.

Box 6.1 A summary of *Good Medical Practice*,[2] which sets out the principles of professional practice

- *Providing good clinical care*: practise good standards of clinical care within the limits of your ability; make sure patients are not put at unnecessary risk.
- *Maintaining good medical practice*: keep updated with developments, skills and indemnity cover.
- *Relationships with patients*: develop, encourage and maintain trust, confidentiality, communication and successful relationships with your patients.
- *Working with colleagues*: work effectively with colleagues, other healthcare professionals and allied healthcare workers.
- *Teaching and training, appraising and assessing*: develop the skills, attitudes and practices to be competent at each.
- *Probity*: be honest at all times.
- *Health*: maintain your health and ensure your own health does not put anybody at risk.

SKILLS

The essential skills that graduates need must be gained under supervision. Medical schools must assess students' competence in these skills.[1]

Graduates from medical school must be competent in various general skills (*see* Box 6.2). Some of these skills are tested, practised and illustrated by various elements of the undergraduate medical degree course. *Tomorrow's Doctors*[1] contains a list of the clinical and practical skills required of a graduate medical student. Familiarise yourself with these in order to ensure you gain plenty of experience during your undergraduate training.

COURSES ON OFFER

UK undergraduate medical courses range from four to six years in length. An overview of a 'typical medical course' is impossible because medical schools in the UK are free to develop their own courses and assessments providing they conform to the GMC recommendations.[3] To find details of particular courses look on the institution's website and in its prospectus.

All medical courses comprise two main components: core and options.[4] The compulsory core component comprises about two-thirds of the whole degree and

> **Box 6.2 Skills required in medical school graduates that are tested, practised and illustrated by various elements of the course structure**[1]
> - *Time management* of self and others
> - Effective *prioritisation* of tasks
> - *Reflection* of practice and work
> - *Problem-solving* in clinical and non-clinical work
> - *Decision-making* and *judgement*
> - *Health promotion* and public health
> - Understanding of *ethics* and *law*
> - Effective and useful *communication*

is primarily undertaken in a problem-based learning (PBL) style or as a didactic, lecture-based course; many courses use elements of both. Within the core curriculum, learning occurs in different settings, that is, within university buildings and clinical settings. The core component encompasses not just clinical knowledge, but the skills, attitudes and behaviour that you are expected to demonstrate as a doctor.[4] The options component of the course mainly comprises Student Selected Components (SSCs) or Student Selected Modules (SSMs) (*see* Chapter 15) and the elective (*see The Medical Student's Survival Guide 2: going clinical*), although different medical schools will incorporate other options-based components, for example research projects.

If you do not think you will be working in clinical medicine when you qualify, you are still expected to achieve all the curriculum outcomes in order to qualify. Medical schools must produce doctors who are fit for clinical practice. If you choose to do something different after you graduate, this is your decision and does not alter the requirements for your graduation.[4]

Systems-based versus subject-based courses

Courses are described as 'systems-based' or 'subject-based'. Systems-based courses are those that teach you medicine in modules that are based on a body 'system'; for example, the gastrointestinal system (from mouth to anus plus liver and pancreas), nervous system (brain, spinal cord and peripheral nerves), cardiovascular system (heart, blood vessels and blood) and so on. Modules contain basic anatomy, physiology (how each organ/system works), histology (looking at cells and tissues), microbiology (learning about the organisms that can damage or help the system), pathology (how things go wrong in the system), pharmacology (drugs that can be used and how they work) and so on. Systems-based courses provide a clinically relevant environment in which to learn the basic sciences.

Subject-based courses are becoming less popular in the advent of PBL. This type of course comprises modules that just cover the anatomy or physiology and so forth of every system all at once. You are learning the processes and techniques of each subject rather than how the body systems work as a whole.

Despite many courses moving towards systems-based teaching, some may still examine subjects (e.g. anatomy) separately to ensure basic science knowledge is solid. Make sure you quickly understand how your medical school will teach and examine you.

Vertical themes

'Vertical themes' are themes, topics or concepts that are so important in medical practice that they keep recurring throughout the years you are studying medicine. Vertical themes will include communication skills, ethics and evidence-based medicine.

Course length

The standard medicine degree takes five or six years. Six-year courses may include graduation in a Bachelor of Science degree after three years, or a pre-medical course (for those who had inadequate grades for direct entry). An additional year may be included for those who choose to intercalate (*see below*). Four-year courses are available for graduate students at some medical schools.

Graduate courses

The four-year graduate courses are not offered by all medical schools and are often only available to students whose first degrees are in biological science. Graduate courses usually require a medical science-related degree to be passed at least at a 2:1 level. Appropriate degrees may include life sciences, bioscience, dentistry, biochemistry, pharmacology and physiology. In addition, graduate students will be required to hold a suitable combination of A levels (or equivalent) at good grades (e.g. at least grades B, B and C or above).

The early academic years in a graduate course are longer than those of the five-year course to enable more to be covered. Often, the first two years' work from a traditional five-year course is squashed into the first year of a graduate programme.

Intercalated degrees

An intercalated degree is a one-year degree course that can be undertaken during a year away from your medical degree. Subjects available to study often include ana-tomical science, biochemistry, cellular and molecular pathology, history of medicine, microbiology, molecular biology, pathology, pharmacology and physiology.

Intercalated degrees are usually undertaken at the end of Year 2, 3 or 4. Although some universities expect all students to undertake an intercalated degree, in many medical schools you have to apply to undertake the degree. If you have to apply to do an intercalated degree, the selection process is based on academic ability, interest and enthusiasm. Students who are drawn to intercalated degrees are usually more interested in medical research and practise deep and strategic learning.[5]

Usually research-based, intercalated degrees will provide you with ample opportunity to learn how to critically evaluate research papers. You may get the chance to experience laboratory-based research and gain practice at writing a scientific paper. These are all skills that you may require in your future career.

Intercalated degrees provide you with a good additional qualification on your CV and in future job applications. However, if undertaking an intercalated degree is the norm for your medical school, the fact that you have done so may not be recognised unless you also gained a high grade or a publication in a well-respected journal.

If you think this would interest you in the future, check in the university prospectus, or contact the university before you apply, to see if it offers this option.

PROBLEM-BASED LEARNING

⫸   **The emphasis is on learning rather than teaching.**

PBL was widely introduced in response to the GMC statement that 'factual information must be kept to the essential minimum that students need at this stage of medical education'.[1] PBL refers to small group (eight to ten members) learning that is based upon identification of knowledge deficits, discussion and study of learning objectives derived from a given, often written, clinical scenario. In some cases trigger media for discussion, such as photographs, journal articles or newspaper clippings are used.[6]

You are expected to read the scenario as a group, defining unknown or unfamiliar words and ensuring all members understand the case. Next, identify important pieces of information ('cues', 'triggers'), within the scenario that require explanation or expansion. Once the cues have been found, the group links information together to formulate hypotheses to describe the case.

While formulating hypotheses you will discover gaps in your knowledge, and these should be noted down as group-agreed 'learning objectives'. In addition to gaps in knowledge arising from the hypotheses, students should set learning objectives for the underlying basic clinical sciences of the case, the normal structure and function of the organ system involved and the psychosocial issues that are raised. The learning objectives, often written in the form of a question, are the basis of your study in preparation for the next session. At the second session, each member of the group should participate in a discussion of the knowledge obtained in response to each learning objective.

Some courses provide a third session in a week. If present, the third session should be used to discuss knowledge gaps or uncertainties arising from the second session.

In the pre-clinical years, you primarily learn about the normal structure and function of systems. However, if your medical school continues PBL into the clinical years, the basic, norm-based knowledge is developed further and you will investigate the ways in which the body can go wrong and become diseased. In addition, clinical experience can be brought into the discussion and management plans may be formulated.

Each week a different case is discussed, and with each new case a new chair and scribe are appointed to lead the group and write the notes, respectively. The chair should ensure a good, directed discussion, that all the important information is covered and that every group member contributes. The scribe should write down the important cues, formulated links and hypotheses. As learning objectives are agreed the scribe writes these down to ensure the group members all work to the same aims.

A tutor/facilitator who is qualified in basic sciences or medicine is appointed to each group, but often only participates in the discussion if the students are fundamentally wrong or missing something. In addition, the tutor may intervene if the group becomes quiet or a deeper understanding should be demonstrated. The knowledge of the tutor can be drawn upon if uncertainty or misunderstanding occurs within the group.

Advantages
Student directed
PBL encourages deeper learning by stimulating interest.[7] The process of investigation of appropriate information teaches skills that can be used in life-long learning/continuing medical education, which is crucial for being a good doctor.[7]

Encourages reflection
PBL requires you to learn independently. Subsequent discussions that take place with your peers will assist you to evaluate your information-gathering skills as well as the depth of the knowledge you have obtained. This encourages reflection on your learning skills and leads to development of more effective strategies.

Improves communication and explanation skills
PBL provides an opportunity to practise technical and lay explanations. Discussions with your peers and tutors will utilise both types of language. In addition, such group work teaches invaluable team-working[7] skills as you endeavour to reach the common goal of finding answers and sharing knowledge. Ideally, such interaction in PBL cultivates an enjoyable learning experience for the students and the tutor.[7]

Improves integration of basic and applied clinical sciences from an earlier stage[8]
As a result of the systems-based learning method that PBL encourages (*see above*)

you will gain an integrated knowledge of basic sciences and clinical work. The relevance of some topics is more obvious and thus information is better retained.

Enhanced critical thinking ability

Students undertaking PBL-based courses develop improved critical thinking ability compared to students taught on lecture-based courses.[9] PBL is also thought to improve self-confidence and self-efficacy, which in turn improves motivation.[9]

Disadvantages

Complicated at the beginning

Group dynamics may not be effective from the start. PBL involves many processes, and newcomers may find each step difficult and the transition between the steps artificial. However, each group usually soon settles into a routine that works best for its members (with/without guidance from the tutor).

Not always clear about depth and breadth of knowledge to be covered

Medicine is a vast subject; you could study the smallest topic for a year and still find new information. Thus it is often difficult to know how much to cover for each learning objective. This difficulty also translates into revision. Although you are never certain, the depth of knowledge required becomes more obvious as you become more experienced. Your tutor should prompt you if deeper discussion is required.

Not suited to those with poor motivation (but neither is being a doctor)

If you find it difficult to sit down and work because everything else always seems more important every time you think about opening a textbook, PBL probably is not for you. You may need the 'spoon-fed' information of a didactic course to *make* you learn. This is fine; just make sure you choose your medical school appropriately. Rarely will anyone find every aspect of medicine interesting; however, if you really cannot be bothered to work at all, think about whether it is PBL that is not for you or being a doctor? There is hard work and a lot of stress ahead of you, if motivation for learning is not there at an early stage you may struggle to keep up as you continue through your course and career.

Associated with worse basic science knowledge[7]

Although this is not unanimously proven, PBL is associated with worse basic science knowledge than older styles of courses. If you really like the idea of a PBL course, just make sure you concentrate on your basic sciences and ask for help whenever you get stuck. You will not end up worse than others if you put the effort in. PBL is specifically associated with poorer anatomy knowledge than that gained through a lecture-based course. With the reduced body donors and subsequent removal of dissection from some medical school curricula, you must make a special effort to work hard on learning your anatomy. If dissection is not available, it is not the end of the world, there are always operating theatres to learn in.

Not suited to some medical students' attitudes

Medical school breeds competition in already competitive people. PBL does not always work well because some members do not like to share their knowledge for fear of empowering the 'competition'. Respect for colleagues is an aim of PBL (and a requirement of the GMC). Blatant demonstrations of disrespect should be disciplined to prevent shattering of confidence. If you encounter problem students, try and address this as a group or have a word with your tutor.

PBL is not respected by all

Some medical students and doctors can be guilty of not respecting the PBL process. This has the effect of undermining the benefits of this type of course and results in the process not being as useful.

Individual needs can be overridden by group learning needs[7]

You will all have different backgrounds. Schools teach their A levels in different ways, and other people may have done degrees or subjects you have not. This can result in a large variation in learning needs. Combat this by undertaking personal study in your lacking areas before the first session (if the cases are available to you in advance) or during the allotted study week for each case. You must meet all set learning objectives; however, feel free to devise your own to meet your learning needs.

LECTURE-BASED COURSES

Often referred to as 'didactic learning', the traditional lecture-based courses delineate exactly what you need to know. Lecture-based courses are well on their way to extinction; however, many courses still incorporate lectures into their curriculum to some extent. Find out what proportion of the medical course at your favourite university is delivered using lectures and thus whether that course will suit your learning style.

> Due to the graphic nature of many of the presentations, subjects of a weak disposition should look away . . . or definitely not attempt to stuff yourself until you are well accustomed to the images that are about to be unleashed onto your brainstem vomiting centre. Some lectures may be as basic and to the point as 'Pus – a clinical view', where you are taken through the huge variety of, talked through the different generations

and generally bombarded with image after image of the exciting world of bodily oozes. *(Elizabeth Li, second-year medical student, Manchester)*

Lecture-based courses are not designed to totally spoon-feed you. Study the subject before the lecture and cover any parts you found difficult afterwards. Medical student Paul White provides some advice for getting the most out of lectures in Box 6.3.

Box 6.3 How to get the most out of lectures (Paul White, second-year medical student, St Andrews)
- Prepare by reading up on the topic beforehand
- Associate what you have learnt with other aspects of the day (e.g. the weather that day or an event) so that you can recall it at a later date
- Ask questions – you are probably not the only one who does not understand
- After the lecture, consolidate your new knowledge by organising your notes alongside any other notes you have written on the subject; read up on the subject using textbooks or the internet and ensure you understand everything
- Make good lecture notes so you do not have to rewrite them later, as this can waste time

Advantages
Lectures provide a good overview
A lecture may introduce you to a topic which you are greatly interested in. This will inspire you to gather further information and knowledge afterwards.

Lectures are perfect for those of you with photographic memories
If you only need to see something once to remember it, and understand it the first time round, lectures will teach you well.

You will be clear about what you are expected to know
Even if the content of the lecture does not contain the depth required, your lecturer will often signpost you to the amount of information you are required to learn.

You will get up-to-the-minute information
Lecturers will often speak about information gained from the most recent research. This will be more relevant than information published in a textbook, which can often be out of date.

Disadvantages
You can be exposed to bias

Lecturers, just like doctors in clinical practice, often have their own ideas, views or interpretation of research or information. Therefore, if your main source of information on a particular topic arises from one lecturer, your learning may be inappropriately biased. If you are on a lecture-based course, remember to remain open minded to other sources of information of differing views, opinions or interpretations.

It can be hard to maintain adequate concentration through an entire lecture

Your concentration will wane throughout a period of an hour, no matter how interested you are in the topic. Therefore, you run the risk of missing crucial explanations or facts.

You have to keep up

Some concepts are more difficult than others. Some of you may need to cover topics a number of times, from a number of sources, before you understand them. A lecturer will continue regardless, especially if the majority of the audience appear to be following. Therefore, if you do not keep up you may not understand the rest of the lecture.

It can be easy to be lazy

You have been told some or all of a particular topic therefore it can be easy to think you do not need to do any further work. It has already been stated that lectures may not cover the depth of knowledge required so you will not have the knowledge expected of you if you do no further work.

> I really cannot stand people who are always first to ask/answer questions in lectures and never let anyone else get a chance, it is so annoying.
> (Rachel Boyce, third-year medical student, Aberdeen)

SPIRAL CURRICULUM

Medical school curricula may be described as being spiral. This refers to the systems-based courses and explains the process of repeated return to topics as you progress through medical school.

Figure 6.1 illustrates a generic spiral curriculum, based on a five-year course. The first two years are spent covering the body using, in this example, four major systems (this varies between medical schools). The early years are focused on learning normal structure and function of the systems, providing the basis for all future learning and understanding.

In the third and fourth years the same systems are covered again, but knowledge of the normal structure and function is revised while you learn about how the systems go wrong. You will cover common diseases and learn relevant basic clinical skills.

The final year of your course is spent consolidating your knowledge on all the body systems and preparing you for your life as a junior doctor. This final year also incorporates learning about managing acutely and/or seriously ill patients, an area that previous medical students have not been competent in. The key competencies in acute care that you should aim to achieve at medical school were devised via a project, ACUTE, jointly undertaken by the Resuscitation Council (UK) and the Intercollegiate Board for Training in Intensive Care Medicine. These key competencies and details of this project can be found at www.resus.org.uk/acute/projrept.pdf.

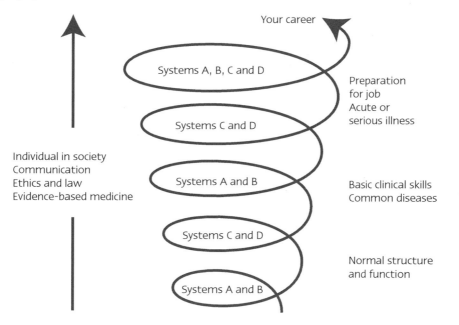

Figure 6.1 The spiral curriculum (adapted from information provided by The University of Manchester School of Medicine).

CLINICAL EXPOSURE

Timing of clinical exposure is different at each medical school. Some medical schools introduce you to patients in your first week. Other medical schools do not offer significant patient contact until year three of a five-year course.

Early 'clinical exposure' sometimes consists of attending nurseries, nursing homes, residential homes or a family containing a pregnant woman, disabled individual or a patient with a chronic illness. In these cases you are expected to follow, either, a particular child, resident or family for a period of time and bring your core knowledge into evaluating them and watching them develop. It also provides you with a chance to practise talking to and gaining rapport with strangers and people of different ages.

> I really like a pre-clinical/clinical divide. This split means you know something when you get on to the wards. Phase one (the pre-clinical years) is clinically oriented, that is, all the science is supported with case studies and clinical scenarios that keep you interested. We do see patients during phase one, but only in a socio-economic/psychosocial sense, rather than for purely medical reasons. (*Zoe Cowan, first-year medical student, Leicester*)

The benefits of early exposure include an obvious correlation between the basic science and the clinical setting. This can improve interest and motivation to learn. Early clinical exposure also benefits those who realise medicine is not for them once they are exposed to the clinical setting. Although this is not a good situation to be in, at least you will know before you have invested too much time and money in the course.[10]

Disadvantages of early clinical exposure may include a lack of confidence. This can result from not having a lot of medical knowledge under your belt when you are meeting patients who instinctively ask medical-related questions. Until you have learnt the basics of clinical history and examination you also cannot obtain a great deal of information from these skills. This may accentuate your already reduced confidence as it can cause confusion when you are asked to present your findings in front of a patient.

Think about when you would want your clinical experience to start and investigate this when deciding which medical school you are interested in, if it is not yet too late.

Inter-professional training

Some courses teach groups that comprise not only medical students but also students training to enter another profession, for example dentistry, nursing or physiotherapy. This can improve your learning experience, as well as your understanding of the roles of each of the different professionals. Hopefully your attitude towards inter-professional collaboration during your future career will be improved.[11]

FURTHER READING

Wood DF. ABC of learning and teaching in medicine: problem based learning. *BMJ*. 2003; **326**: 328–30.

CHAPTER 7

Learning

Hard work pays off in the future. Laziness pays off now.[1]

Everyone is different. Medicine involves pattern recognition, interpretation, identification of inconsistencies and acquisition of many concepts and facts. Early in your degree you must learn how to study efficiently, and what and how much you need to know.

You are responsible for your learning. Organise your time and be proactive in obtaining knowledge. Medical degrees are designed to teach students how to be life-long learners. Self-directed learning does not stop upon graduation. To assist this process, your medical school will provide you with education, training and facilities through which you can achieve an undergraduate medical qualification.[2] Relevant standards have been set out by the Council of Heads of Medical Schools (CHMS) and the British Medical Association Medical Students Committee (BMA MSC) and have been summarised in Appendix III.

Adults are motivated by learning that:[3]
- Is perceived as relevant
- Is based on, and builds on, their previous experience
- Is participatory and actively involves them
- Is focused on problems
- Is designed so that they can take responsibility for their own learning
- Can be immediately applied in practice
- Involves cycles of action and reflection
- Is based on mutual trust and respect.

WHEN

Start working as early as possible. Everything you learn builds upon previously acquired knowledge. Poor foundations will result in future difficulties. In addition, early initiation of work allows time to return to the topics to improve retention of knowledge. Learning is also more effective if it is spread over a long period than if knowledge is 'crammed'.[4]

Only you know when you study best. Are you an early bird or do you like to burn the midnight oil? Discover your preference then study at the time when you are at your most enthusiastic, efficient and industrious. Do not force yourself to work if you are really not in the mood. Plan your study around natural breaks such as sports, activities, a television programme or meal times.

Use any opportunity you can as a learning opportunity

Once you start medical school, all non-medical friends and family look to you for explanations of medical topics in the media and their own health problems. There are three ways of dealing with this.

1. Tell the person that you do not know. You have not yet covered everything.
2. Tell the person who asked that you do not know but will endeavour to find out and get back to them.
3. Be one step ahead. Use each media story/health problem as a learning stimulus and investigate the topic before anyone has chance to ask.

Investigating media medical topics will not just prove to your parents/partner/self that their/your tuition fees are being put to good use, it will also assist you in interviews and exams, in which media 'hot topics' often arise. The media can also demonstrate descriptions of conditions in a 'lay language'. Just make sure you do not adopt the media's sensationalism and bias.

Medical documentaries can be useful for introducing you to certain topics, although you must be wary that the information provided is often not 100% accurate. Indeed, even medical dramas can be a good introduction to some topics. You may be surprised how many times *Casualty* or *ER* is mentioned during a problem-based learning (PBL) session or a medical discussion. You may relate to patients through these programmes as this may be the only previous exposure they have had to a hospital environment/particular medical condition.

WHERE

> Teaching and learning systems must take account of modern educational theory and research, and make use of modern technologies where evidence shows that these are effective.[5]

Where you decide to study is very much dependent on what you are going to learn. Medicine involves a plethora of subjects and there is not one place in which you will be able to master them all.

Independent learning

> I tend to do all my learning either in the library or IT suites, which means when I get home I can switch off. *(Pauline Law, first-year graduate medical student, Dundee)*

Unfortunately, sticking your head in a book is the only way to acquire some of the knowledge required for your medical degree; basic sciences, epidemiology of diseases and literature-based research are some examples. Everybody learns differently (see the 'How' section below); however, you generally have two environments in which to do book work: at home or in the library.

A healthy attitude to work clearly segregates study from relaxation. It can be impossible to 'switch off' when you are sleeping in the same room as your desk and books. Working in a library may be a solution, although libraries have the disadvantages of conversation all around you and time restrictions due to opening hours. Working at your accommodation ensures food and drink are readily available, you know where all your books are and you can play music while you study. Periodically assess your current study environment and decide whether it provides you with the most effective use of time.

University libraries are very comprehensive. They contain a vast variety of books, although not always enough of each. Libraries are increasingly computerised to enable easy searches of library stock or holdings, remote access library accounts to renew and order books and self-service check-in and book return. There is easy access to photocopiers and computers with internet access. Medical students are often privileged with their own medical library.

You have access to laboratories to learn basic science, such as physiology (how the body and its parts work) and histology (looking at cells and tissues under microscopes). However, time is limited and there is an awful lot to learn. To get more than the basic information out of laboratory work, read about the techniques and basic concepts before the practical session. You can then ask your tutors to explain the more difficult or advanced concepts.

Group learning

Group learning is encouraged in courses that use PBL. The PBL process requires small groups to identify, discuss and work through problems together. However, small-group learning can also occur in other settings. Tutorials during clinical placements may occur at the patient's bedside, e.g. learn and practise history and examination techniques, or away from patients, e.g. to discuss a particular case or condition.

Lectures are used to teach large groups and, although it is possible, usually do not consist of a discussion but an outline of key knowledge. The PBL process does not endorse lectures; however, a few lectures may be provided to cover basic knowledge, common areas of uncertainty or rare/interesting cases.

Anatomy

A dissection laboratory contains many bodies, one of which is allocated to each small group and is dissected at regular intervals. Not all medical schools offer dissection. A similar alternative is pre-dissected body 'sections'. These are sometimes made available even in schools offering dissection to demonstrate the anatomy of intricate body parts or those that require much investigation, e.g. arms, abdomen or the head. Dissection provides a wealth of time to investigate and understand anatomical features and relationships. The main criticism of learning anatomy through dissection is that some body structures change appearance, texture and size as a result of the preservation process or simply because they are not in a living body.

Computer-assisted learning (CAL) packages are increasingly sophisticated and are becoming the primary anatomy resource in medical schools that do not undertake dissection. As body imaging also improves, this is combined with computer-based learning. Some medical schools even teach anatomy by superimposing 3D images of the human body components onto the flesh of a living student to demonstrate the relationship, size and position of structures in a clinically relevant way.

Surgery may fill some of the anatomy knowledge gaps you have. Surgeons are the best doctors from whom you can learn anatomy during your clinical years. Use the operating theatre to witness the living, working structures of the body (e.g. the beating heart and peristalsis in the intestines). Organise a session(s) with your local pathologists to watch post-mortems. Post-mortems are carried out to determine the cause of death in the patient. Often this does not comprise complete dissection, but investigation of the appropriate systems until enough information has been gleaned. Depending on the pathologist, the number of students wanting to attend, regulations and facilities, you will either watch from a balcony or at the deceased's side. It is fascinating to observe the close inspection of organs and systems while thinking about the history of the patient. Hypotheses can be made about the mechanisms of death and evidence to support or refute these is sought.

Book-based resources are useful to familiarise yourself with basic anatomy. However, learning all your anatomy like this is not appropriate: you will gain an incomplete understanding and appreciation of the size, relationship and physiology of each structure.

Clinical skills

'Clinical skills' are the practical skills that you perform as a medical student (e.g. taking blood, measuring blood pressure, taking a history). Initially, you will be introduced to clinical skills in a laboratory containing relevant 'plastic-dummies' and facilities for learning and practice. 'Skills labs' may be available for individual or small-group practice throughout term and before exams; ask your skills tutors about availability at your medical school. The problem with skills labs is that, good as the dummies are, they are not entirely realistic. Sometimes they are easier to perform the skill on than real patients and sometimes they are harder, but either way the emotional, patient contact component is never present, this can sometimes be the most difficult aspect of any skill.

Clinical placements, with real patients and real needs for investigations, are the best environment in which to practise your clinical skills. You get to practise your clinical skills while participating in the patient's management. The significance of any skill is more obvious if it is associated with a real-life situation. Healthcare professionals will often be happy to observe, supervise, chaperone or assist you when necessary.

Books can provide the theoretical basis to clinical skills, for example what you need to do and why you are doing it. However, theory is useless without the ability to perform the skill. You will struggle in exams and as a doctor if you cannot perform basic clinical skills when you graduate.

Courses and external lectures

Courses and non-curriculum-based lectures exist for medical students to learn clinical skills. The Royal Colleges often run free or cheap courses to introduce medical students to their specialty. Individual universities, defence organisations and medical-related associations or companies may run local or national skills courses, with varying fees. Keep your eyes and ears open for these courses. Details of skills courses are usually found on medical websites or in medical student journals.

Professional Medical Education

Basic life support – what do you do until the crash team gets there? If you are unsure of how to resuscitate a person from a cardiac arrest, then you at least need to be completely up-to-date with keeping the patient alive until help arrives. Professional Medical Education (PME) runs courses to teach you what to do.

Practical skills – shoulder injections, knee aspiration, catheterisation, central lines; there are a lot of practical procedures we have to undertake on a daily basis, and the time allocated at medical school may not always give you enough experience. Join PME on a practical skills course and you will learn how to suture, splint a fracture and more. See the website (www.freefees.co.uk).

WHAT

> Medicine . . . not a lot is difficult but there is a lot of it.

During medical school, learn all the essential knowledge, skills and attitudes that you require as a junior doctor. By no means are you expected to know everything. Unfortunately this creates difficulty – as an undergraduate you often feel like you do not know enough, yet you never know how much you need to know. Medical schools design their courses to comply with suggested curricular outcomes but it is the student's responsibility to achieve these outcomes.

Advice on the breadth and depth of required knowledge should come from your tutors and lecturers. Universities should provide you with the subject areas, objectives and essential skills you are required to learn during each module. Look through this list at the beginning of the module and slot relevant topics into weekly learning objectives.

Gain solid knowledge and understanding of basic, clinical, behavioural and social sciences, and be able to integrate these sciences to form a good foundation for your career. Learn how lifestyle, genetic, social and environmental factors affect disease occurrence, progression, treatment and prevention. Above all, make sure you understand what you learn:

➡ Do you know the precise definition of terms you are learning?
➡ Can you explain the concept to a non-medical person?
➡ What is the mechanism underlying the phenomenon you have just learnt?

Early in medical school you learn about the normal structure and function of the body. Once you understand normality and the underlying science, working out how things can go wrong is easy. The defence systems of the body, normal variants and reactions to insults are bridges between normal and abnormal body function.[5]

> Factual information must be kept to the essential minimum that students need at this stage of medical education.[5]

Be aware of alternative and complementary therapies. Why do patients use them? How do they influence and interact with more conventional medical treatment? What are the important advantages and disadvantages?[5]

Do not forget about psychosocial concepts. Medical students often groan (or laugh) at this 'touchy feely' subject. However, without covering psychosocial topics you will have no hope of understanding your patients, why they act the way they do or how to help people. Realise the interplay between mental and physical health and how each can directly and indirectly affect the other (Figure 7.1).

Interpret the whole picture

Medicine requires the ability to interpret situations not individual facts. No patients or illnesses present in the same way. Patients often present with more than one symptom or problem. Often, multiple problems have a common cause, rather than each being attributed to different diagnoses. A rigid or narrow approach to assessment, diagnosis and management planning does not accommodate efficient processing of all available information and can lead to inaccurate diagnosis. Even at times when a structured approach to assessment is required (e.g. in emergencies) you should still look at the patient and situation as a whole to gain maximal information and to ensure safety.

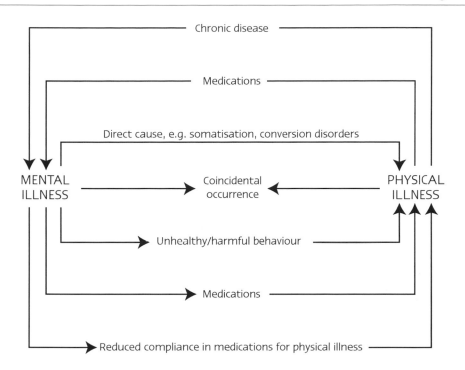

Figure 7.1 Interplay between mental and physical health.

HOW

Learning opportunities must help students explore knowledge, and evaluate and integrate evidence critically. The curriculum must motivate students and help them develop the skills for self-directed learning.[5]

Methods

Deep learning . . . is motivated by a desire for personal understanding and vocational relevance and demonstrated by the student's searching for principles and the integration of knowledge across all different domains.[6]

Learning is a personal process. You cannot be told your best learning method, you have to discover it. However, you can be made aware of the methods that students use to consider your options. Different approaches to learning can be amalgamated and each will have their uses at some point during your course. Evaluate your learning approach for efficiency and efficacy; change it if it is not working for you.

Go back to basics

Medical knowledge has to be solid from the outset. Basic clinical science concepts are crucial foundations for the clinical knowledge you require later in medical school. Do not assume, if you have done A-level biology, that you know all the required basic sciences. Revise or learn the concepts again from the beginning.

You cannot learn all the answers to all the questions that will be thrown at you during your career. However, if you have learnt from basic principles, you can work out answers to most questions.

Patients ask questions about their condition and how their medicines work; you must explain the answers in terms that they can understand. If you have only learnt that their 'cholesterol tablet' is an HMG-CoA reductase inhibitor, but do not know what that means, you are not going to further their understanding of the medication you are asking them to take every day for the rest of their lives.

Repeatedly return to topics

Not all the concepts you learn at medical school will be used on a day to day basis. However, retention for easy recall is necessary for exams and your career. Devise a system whereby you ensure you will regularly return to topics time after time. You can buy multiple choice question books and access questions on line; below are a few ideas to do yourself to create learning and revision tools that are specific to your course and needs.

Convert books and notes into either true/false or open questions. You can write the question on one side of a piece of paper or card and the answer on the other. Keep these questions in a box and, whenever you have a spare minute, go through a few cards. If you get the answer right, put the card at the back of the box; if you get it wrong put it somewhere near the centre of the box to ensure you return to it more quickly than those you know well. Throughout university keep adding to the questions. Eventually your random questions will cover a wide range of topics.

Enzymes

Cell membranes, receptors and ion channels

Identifying and managing cardiovascular risk factors

Normal structure and function of each organ system

Anti-cholinergic side effects

For those of you who are computer-literate, create a slideshow presentation that contains questions and answers. Use the animation function so that only the question is on the screen initially. Once you have considered the answer get the answer to 'pop up' at the click of a button. You can keep adding slides and organise the 'slideshows' into topics.

Writing notes

Most medical students write notes. Notes on textbooks, lectures, tips or information from peers, things that you need to look up and even your own notes. But what are these notes for?

Notes may serve as a reminder of the information you need to study in more depth when you have the chance. However, notes are often written as part of learning and revision as well as for use during these processes.

> I was mocked by one of my tutors for writing notes while in my first year at university. He asked me for how long I intended writing notes, and whether I felt that it was constructive. At the time I was quite shocked. I had always found note-writing to be a useful way of focusing my interest on what I was learning. Although his comments continued to haunt me, I carried on doing it. Subsequently, I have successfully completed medical school, and I cannot say my note-writing was a hindrance at any point. (*Anonymous*)

Notes that summarise information from textbooks clearly demonstrate the important information. Furthermore, different textbooks provide different depths and breadths of knowledge. Thus, notes can collate all available information into one place. Some students take this one step further and use their learning notes to write revision notes, resulting in a vastly abbreviated document of key points.

Some students do not even consult the notes after they have been written – so what is the point? Learning is a personal thing. Some people find it easy to read a passage in a textbook and remember it. Others require a more interactive style of learning. For the latter group, writing notes serves only to provide a focus during bookwork, which is equally acceptable.

Highlighting notes or textbooks

If you find writing notes too time-consuming, you may prefer highlighting important concepts in textbooks. This enables you to return to the textbook in the future and quickly pick out the important information.

This approach does not work for those students who have a 'thing' about writing in books. In addition, if you are planning to sell your books once you are finished with them, this approach will greatly reduce their value. In addition, as you progress through medical school, some information that was initially new and important becomes second nature. If you highlighted these basic points they may later detract from the crucial information in the future. An alternative to highlighting textbooks is to write notes initially and then highlight the important information in your notes.

> Getting down to doing work – highlight and annotate textbooks! Buy the bare essential, core, brilliant books (probably an anatomy and physiology) and attack it with all the colours of the rainbow. If it's not beyond your battered brain's abilities, attempt some sort of colour-coding. Then move on to a more complex book (pure physiology, for example) and add any extra 'This will get me a gold star' bits and bobs on the side of your already highlighted book. Basically, this is a cheat that gives you a great set of notes without the trawl of actually writing them out, plus you've already picked out the relevant juicy bits. Saves a VAST amount of time and you're able to get through more material. (*Elizabeth Li, second-year medical student, Manchester*)

List learning

Many medical students learn lists. Although criticised for causing students to learn and recite knowledge 'parrot fashion', lists can have their uses. Some information in medicine cannot be worked out and does just have to be learned. But be careful. If you are learning information on one topic, list-learning can be a quick and easy way to get through the information. You can cram lists into your head in preparation for a discussion or exam the next day, but then what happens? You will probably forget it. As you progress through medical school you will have to relearn the lists, which will be increasingly difficult as you accumulate increasing amounts of 'dry' information.

In its true form, list learning is referred to as involving 'dry' information because no calculation has been used to reach the information. You are literally just learning a sequence of words. In reality, however, list-learners are probably using basic knowledge to help them remember the contents of the list.

Do be careful if you are a list-learner. You may find it difficult to answer abstract questions, that is, those that are related to knowledge you have learnt but not directly linked to it. If you have not learnt how the contents of your list are related, you will find problem-solving and non-typical presentations of illnesses awkward. List-learning cramming for revision will not be possible if you have general exams that cover all aspects of medicine.

Mnemonics and acronyms

Although commonly used, mnemonics and acronyms are usually not useful for primary learning. They do not represent a basic understanding. Acronyms are used to name drug trials, to describe procedures and diagnoses, and to name organisations.

Historically, medical professionals used acronyms to speak about patients in a derogatory way without being found out, for example BUNDY ('but unfortunately not dead yet'). In an increasingly politically correct and litigious environment, such use of acronyms is totally unacceptable. Even medical or procedural-based acronyms should be avoided as some have multiple meanings, depending on the specialty in which they are used; this can cause confusion and errors.

> Signs of shock = SHOCKS
> ➡ Sinus tachycardia
> ➡ Hypotension
> ➡ Oliguria
> ➡ Cold
> ➡ Klammy(!)
> ➡ Slow capillary refill. *(Dr Bob Clarke)*

Despite all their criticisms, mnemonics and acronyms can assist recall of information, especially during management of an emergency situation; the easy recall that mnemonics provides helps you to remember information under pressure. For example, main components of the treatment of a heart attack, MONA (morphine, oxygen, nitrates and aspirin). Obviously you still need to know the full management, but this will get you started.

Aside from emergencies, mnemonics or acronyms can be useful during other situations in which you are nervous. For example, when taking a history of a presenting complaint, SOCRATES will help you to remember the features to ask about (site, onset, character, radiation, associated features, timing, exacerbating/alleviating factors, severity).

Use acronyms and mnemonics to assist recall under pressure but ensure you learn the knowledge underlying the information contained in them as well; DO NOT write them in medical notes.

Surgical sieve

How many times have you been asked 'What are the causes of condition X?' in your clinical years? Not there yet? A good estimate is daily. Because of its frequency you would think every medical student should be able to answer this question easily and with logic. You would be wrong.

The perfect answer to the question 'What are the causes of condition X?' starts with 'The three most common causes are . . . x y z'. Therefore, the first thing you should do, when learning about a condition, is to learn the three most common causes. This is really a 'list-learning' exercise.

The next step is to state further causes of condition X, which is when a logical, structured approach is essential; this is achieved by use of a 'surgical sieve'. The surgical sieve is a template through which you categorise the causes of individual conditions. Examples of the categories used are in Box 7.1. These categories can be remembered using a mnemonic. Feel free to make up your own categories, this order of the categories is not important; being consistent is.

Box 7.1 Pathological categories comprising a surgical sieve
- Iatrogenic (caused by the actions of the medical profession)
- Neoplastic – benign or malignant 'growths'
- Vascular – including blood and heart
- Endocrine (i.e. hormones)
- Structural or mechanical
- Trauma or accident
- Inflammatory
- Genetic or congenital
- Autoimmune
- Toxic
- Infective
- Old age or degenerative
- Nutritional or metabolic
- Spontaneous or idiopathic

The surgical sieve for headache is illustrated below using the categories in Box 7.1 (not all categories will be filled in for each symptom or disease):
➥ Iatrogenic: blood pressure-lowering drugs, lumbar puncture
➥ Neoplastic: benign and malignant brain tumours
➥ Vascular: migraine, cerebrovascular accident
➥ Endocrine: hypoglycaemia
➥ Structural or mechanical: tension headache
➥ Trauma or accident: head injury
➥ Inflammatory: encephalitis
➥ Genetic or congenital
➥ Autoimmune: vasculitis
➥ Toxic: carbon monoxide poisoning
➥ Infective: meningitis (viral, bacterial)
➥ Old age or degenerative: cervical spondylosis
➥ Nutritional or metabolic: dehydration
➥ Spontaneous or idiopathic.

Dancing

You may be surprised to see 'dancing' as a way of learning; however, it can be an effective way of making information memorable. Dr Bob Clarke (www. askdoctorclarke.com) uses a dance in his final year revision course to help medical students remember the ECG features of abnormal potassium levels. It has to be seen to be believed, but it makes the information incredibly memorable.

Sayings or rhymes

> I always used to confuse the opposite effects of parathyroid and calcitonin. The only way I got this knowledge to stick was to remember 'calciton-in-bone', that is, calcitonin puts the calcium in bone. Probably sounds stupid to everyone else but me, but I have not been confused about this again.
> *(Lizzie Cottrell, fifth-year medical student, Manchester)*

Sayings, stories or rhymes can aid your recall of information. For example, the rhyme 'bones, stones, groans and psychic moans' is a perfect reminder of the symptoms of high levels of calcium in the blood.[7]

Rhymes and sayings have been used for a long time. In *The Surgeon's Rhyme*, Dr Barrie recalls a surgeon teacher from medical school who taught them a rhyme to use to answer any question starting with 'What are the causes of . . . [condition X]'. Barrie describes the surgeon becoming angry, any time that the medical students did not follow the rhyme. Although anger is not necessarily constructive, the principle was right, the medical students were being taught to be logical and consistent in order to not miss anything.

Associated learning

Try associating actions or situations with words or concepts in order to improve recall and retention of knowledge. For example, for the word 'supination' (e.g. turning the hand palm up, the opposite of pronation), you can associate supination with a bowl of soup. 'Soup'-ination thus becomes synonymous with turning your hand with the palm uppermost to make the shape you make when you are holding a bowl of soup.

Teach or explain

If you cannot teach or explain the concept you are learning, you do not know it. As a doctor you will not be reciting textbooks to patients, you will need to explain diagnoses and treatments in simple terms. Practise this to ensure that you really understand the information you are learning (your communication skills will also improve).

Practise on medical student friends

Medical students are all striving to reach the same goal. So why don't you practise practical procedures and examinations on each other (when appropriate)? You can take turns being patient, examiner and student, and critique each other's performance within these roles. You will learn from each other and will gain confidence in performing clinical skills under observation.

Keep asking until you understand

Some concepts stump many students, for example, electrocardiogram (ECG; electrical tracing of the heart) interpretation. Sometimes concepts need to be explained in a certain way before you can understand them. If you ask for help from one person and you do not understand, keep asking different people until it is explained in a way that makes sense to you.

Revision resources

Described in more depth in Chapter 8, revision resources (including books, past papers, practice questions and internet-based tutorials and questions) can validate your learning and will ensure that you have covered the salient points. Make sure you choose those most suited to your course. Ask for recommendations from your university and peers.

Use your own experiences

Having experience of being a patient can be incredibly useful in your medical training; however, do not intentionally maim or infect yourself to get this experience. Being a patient makes you aware of patients' priorities and concerns, and what investigations and treatments actually feel like. It is easy for a reassuring medical student to say 'just a small scratch' for something which is exquisitely painful. Use any experience you have of being a patient in your training to educate your peers and yourself.

Resources

Throughout medical school you will use a huge variety of resources. Medicine contains over 60 specialties, numerous areas of expertise and conflicting opinions. Learn how to source and evaluate all relevant information. Learn also about a variety of non-medical subjects. For example, a patient with epilepsy must be advised about whether or not they should drive; for this you need to obtain information from the DVLA. Another example occurs in forensic psychiatry, for which you need to know some law, in addition to general psychiatry, to manage the patients.

This section cannot cover every useful resource. However, it will alert you to the idea that many sources of information exist and through which channels you might obtain this information.

Computer-based learning

Computers are invaluable in the learning environment. Programs, intranet and internet sites are all being developed with education in mind. Computer-aided learning (CAL) packages are available on various topics at most medical schools. CAL packages may consist of a tutorial, a source of reference or an interactive learning module. Those of you who are computer literate can learn by creating CAL packages for your peers to use. Ask your medical school's computer technician or librarian about the CAL packages available for you.

Web-based resources

Readily available internet access is invaluable. There are so many fantastic web-based resources on the internet that you would be really missing out if you did not try them. On discovery of a good website, make a note of it or add it to your 'favourites' folder to help you to find it easily next time.

BMJ Learning

BMJ Learning supports doctors' learning. It is an evidence-based, interactive and continually updated website that has material for junior and senior hospital doctors and general practitioners. BMJ Learning models its resources on the key steps in learning (*see* Box 7.2). Learning modules refer you to national guidelines and list further relevant, useful resources. When you have completed a module, reflect on it to ensure your learning is effective and durable. 'Just-in-time' modules provide bite-sized chunks of learning; 'read reflect respond' modules guide you through ethical or professionalism issues; and 'interactive case histories' test your baseline knowledge, present interactive cases to update your knowledge and then test your post-module knowledge to discover what you have learnt. Over 250 modules are available on the BMJ Learning website, which is continually improving and expanding. To register with BMJ Learning you will need to know your BMA membership number and the postcode to which your paper *BMJ* is sent; see the website www.bmjlearning.com.

Box 7.2 Steps in learning and how BMJ Learning can help (from www. bmjlearning.com)

- *Define* your learning needs
- *Plan* your learning: What do you need to learn? Which resources will you use?
- *Learn*: use BMJ Learning modules that use a range of resources to suit different learning styles
- *Reflect* on what you have learnt. This makes your learning more effective and lasting. What have you learnt? How can you apply your learning to your work? How will you confirm the information has been learnt and retained?

Besttreatments

The BMJ group helped to develop besttreatments.co.uk. This website (www. besttreatments.co.uk) is designed for patients and doctors to get quick and easy information on many different conditions.

eMedicine

The eMedicine website (www.emedicine.com) contains a large clinical knowledge base which is available to healthcare professionals. The evidence-based content is updated regularly and provides best practice guidelines for many medical specialties. The site is easy to search and the information is organised in a useful and consistent way. Learning and resource centres within the site provide continuing medical education, although a charge may apply in some cases.

GPnotebook

GPnotebook (www.gpnotebook.com), an online encyclopaedia of medicine, is an excellent 'first port of call' for clinical information. The information on presentation, investigations, diagnosis and management of many conditions is searchable, succinct and supported by research.

Flesh and bones

The flesh and bones website (www.fleshandbones.com) offers such a fantastic range of learning resources you will wonder if you will ever need to go anywhere else to study. The site contains free chapters from many textbooks. The revision centre provides interactive quizzes, tips, mnemonics and important revision topics. There is an online bookshop, survival guides covering many of the main specialties and games to spend your rest time playing. It is really worth a visit.

Wikipedia

Wikipedia (www.wikipedia.org) is an online encyclopaedia in many different languages. This resource is rapidly growing and, among other information, you can find simple explanations of many medical conditions and the origins of the names of these conditions.

ECG library

Examples and explanations of normal and abnormal ECGs are found at the *ECG library* (www.ecglibrary.com/ecghome.html). The website supports the book *ECGs by Example*,[8] and thus contains corrections, comments and additional information for the book.

Doctors.net.uk

Access to Doctors.net.uk (www.doctors.net.uk) requires free registration. This website provides forums for discussion and a 'library' through which you can perform searches and view online textbooks. The website also contains revision resources, up-to-date medical-related news and a 'free time' area that provides details of weather, TV listings, travel information and various other non-medical related useful resources.

Merck manuals

A wide source of medical information can be found at Merck manuals online (www. merck.com/pubs/), through which you can access *The Merck Manual, The Merck*

Manual of Diagnosis and Therapy, *The Merck Manual of Health and Aging* and *The Merck Manual of Geriatrics*. These searchable, online texts are an excellent and quick source of information.

University of Washington Department of Medicine

The University of Washington, Department of Medicine has a clinical skills section on its website (http://depts.washington.edu/physdx/skillmodules.html). This contains excellent explanations and demonstrations of histories, examinations and investigations. Audio and video clips can be downloaded to enrich your learning. All clinical medical students must visit this website.

NeuroLogic

Worried about your neurology knowledge? NeuroLogic (http://medstat.med. utah.edu/neurologicexam/html/home_exam.html) contains movies, tutorials and interactive quizzes on various aspects of neurology. You can first learn how to perform neurological examinations, the underlying explanations for each examination and reasons for specific findings.

Instant anatomy

The *instant anatomy* website (www.instantanatomy.net) has been developed by Robert Whitaker, a retired surgeon. The website contains audio-visual lectures as well as annotated diagrams, covering a wide range of anatomy. A CD can be purchased from the site and contains tutorials and information in addition to that found on the website.

Trauma.org

Trauma.org (www.trauma.org) is designed to provide global education, information and communication for professionals in trauma and critical care. As the website is not intended for use by the general public, it contains healthcare professional-targeted information. Trauma.org contains an image bank of trauma images and interactive moulages that allow you to work through a trauma situation and get immediate feedback on the answers you provide on the management.

Medical school resources

All medical students should have access to appropriate learning resources and facilities; including libraries, computers (including email, intranet and internet), photocopiers, lecture theatres and seminar rooms. Universities should review the quality of these resources and facilities and ensure they are updated when appropriate.

As a student you have responsibilities for the resources provided by your medical school. Treat all facilities and resources with respect. Should you find a resource or facility to be damaged, broken or incomplete you must report this. Finally, medical students are in the optimum position to state which learning resources and facilities are most needed. If you identify a potentially useful resource that is unavailable, inform your tutors.

Books

> He who studies medicine without books sails an uncharted sea, but he who studies medicine without patients does not go to sea at all. (*Sir William Osler*)[9]

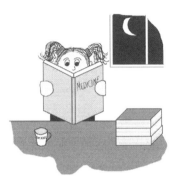

Textbooks feature strongly in undergraduate medical education. They are accessible and easy to use. Before you buy any textbooks, borrow them from the library to ensure they suit your learning style. You will have strong preferences with regard to the style of textbook that you learn well from. It is a waste of money to buy a book that does not conform to these preferences. Good as they are, remember that textbooks are always out of date by the time they are published. Providing you are aware of this you can supplement what you read with information from your tutors, guidelines and research publications. It can also be useful to update the main text (with pencil or sticky notes) with newly published information and facts.

> So far I have bought four textbooks, but I wish I hadn't bothered as I often end up carrying them to the library to work from, only to find there are plenty of copies there. (*Laura Stevens, first-year medical student, Dundee*)

Your university gives you a reading list that you should take notice of: exam questions are often derived from recommended texts. However, beware of textbooks that are written by lecturers or tutors from your university, these may not be the best textbooks around. There is a financial (and ego boosting) incentive for your tutors to encourage you to buy their own books. Sample chapters may help you discover which textbooks match your preferred style. Visit www.fleshandbones.com for a large variety of sample chapters.

> Do not run out and buy books in advance. I have survived quite well on purchasing one really good anatomy book (recommended by my lecturer) and borrowing all the rest from the library. It helps to get to know your library very quickly – and find out how to reserve books that come up on reading lists. Only invest hard cash in something that you will use

all the way through the course. The Medical Students Union will usually organise used book sales, and don't forget to check out notice boards and local Oxfam shops for used copies on an individual basis. *(Pauline Law, first-year graduate medical student, Dundee)*

Below are listed textbooks (or series of textbooks) recommended by medical students around the country. But, remember, no matter how good it is one textbook will never suit all. Medical student Paul White gives information on how to use a textbook in Box 7.3.

General medicine

➡ Crash course series. The Crash Course books were recommended by Rachel Boyce (first-year medical student, Aberdeen). Books are available for most undergraduate topics. Although they are not in-depth texts, they provide a brief overview of the basic and clinical sciences associated with each topic and have practice questions at the end to test your learning.

➡ Kumar P, Clark M. *Clinical Medicine*. 6th ed. Edinburgh: Saunders; 2005. Often referred to as 'the bible' by medical students around the country, Rachel Boyce also recommended the 'Kumar and Clark' website (www.kumarandclark. com). However, Anna Kieslich (fifth-year medical student, Dundee) criticised it for having varying quality from chapter to chapter.

➡ Master Medicine series. Anna Kieslich recommended the Master Medicine series because they are 'basic' and 'easy to understand'. She and Nat Bradbrook (fifth-year medical student, Manchester) felt that the series made concepts easier during early clinical training. The books in this series have a variety of practice questions at the end of each chapter.

➡ Oxford Handbook series. Many books are available in the Oxford Handbook series, including the *Oxford Handbook of Clinical Medicine* and the *Oxford Handbook of Clinical Specialties*. Rachel Boyce recommended the series as a whole and Nat Bradbrook referred to the *Oxford Handbook of Clinical Medicine* as 'the medics' bible'. Being just the right size for a lab coat pocket, there is never any excuse to be far from a short summary of the signs, symptoms and management of many common (and less common) disorders. Do not learn solely from the Oxford Handbooks but use them regularly for reference in the clinical setting.

Anatomy and physiology

➡ Anatomy and physiology colouring-in books. Various anatomy and physiology colouring books are available. Katie Thorne (second-year medical student, York, Hull) recommended these books because they are 'amazing' and 'definitely helped me pass my first-year exams'. These books make you learn without realising it.

➡ Guyton AC, Hall JE. *Textbook of Medical Physiology.* 11th ed. Philadelphia: WB Saunders; 2006. 'Guyton' is an in-depth text but its short sections make it easy to learn from. Copious illustrations improve understanding of the content.

➡ Martini FH. *Fundamentals of Anatomy and Physiology.* 7th ed. Benjamin-Cummings Pub Co; 2005. The basis of many medical students' pre-clinical years. It is simple and superficial in places but a great introduction for new students (and senior students who need to revise basic anatomy and physiology for their finals!).

➡ Moore KL, Dalley AF. *Clinically Oriented Anatomy.* Lippincott Williams & Wilkins; 2005. Laura Stevens (first-year medical student, Dundee) called this book 'the bible'.

Miscellaneous

➡ ABC series. The *British Medical Journal* (BMJ) publishing company publishes the books in the ABC series. The ABC series covers individual specialties ranging from intensive care to rheumatology. They are informative and concise.

➡ Ellis P. *A Companion to ENT for Medical Students and General Practitioners.* Revised 3rd ed. Cambridge: BluePoint Cambridge Ltd; 2001. An excellent overview of the basics of ear, nose and throat (ENT). It is chatty so is easy to read. Topics are described simply so the information is easily understood and retained. In addition, this book suggests appropriate clinical environments in which you may experience the conditions being described.

➡ Lissauer T, Clayden G. *Illustrated Textbook of Paediatrics.* 2nd ed. Edinburgh: Mosby; 2001. A clear and colourful book that is easy to read. The content of this book outlines the required undergraduate paediatric knowledge. A revision book has been written to complement this textbook.

➡ Rang HP, Dale MM, Ritter JM. *Pharmacology.* 5th ed. Edinburgh: Churchill Livingstone; 2003. This pharmacology book probably covers far more information than undergraduates need; however, many students use 'Rang, Dale and Ritter'. It discusses drug groups but also describes the 'stories' behind the development of the drugs and conditions for which they are used.

➡ Underwood JCE. *General and Systematic Pathology.* 4th ed. Edinburgh: Churchill Livingstone; 2004. This book is full of illustrations/photographs which makes it very easy to understand. It is a fantastic introduction and will probably fulfil your pathology needs during your undergraduate medical education.

Journals

A journal is a publication that contains articles, comments and information that targets a particular group of individuals (e.g. medical students, foundation doctors) or specialty (e.g. cardiology, public health). Hundreds of medical journals exist. So what can they offer you?

> **Box 7.3 How to use a textbook (Paul White, second-year medical student, St Andrews)**
> - Focus on key words
> - Read selectively, for example read to find answers to specific questions or learning objectives
> - Break it down into manageable chunks and focus on just one of these at a time; stop and summarise each chunk before proceeding; analyse it, ask questions and check that it is OK
> - Stick to lecture content or learning objectives
> - Survey skim; first, distinguish what you already know; fill in any gaps; and compare with other information that you have already learnt

Journals provide focused and deep information. The information is up-to-the-minute as it is detailing recent or future developments or arises directly from research. Reading journals will keep you updated with the constantly changing world of medicine. This is important in clinical practice as well as during job applications.

> The *StudentBMJ* is easy to read and becomes really relevant in the clinical years. It covers everything from education to what is going on with medical students around the world. It has got a great website. You can also try your hand at writing a piece for it. *(Kate Fraser, fourth-year medical student, Manchester)*

Start reading journals early in your medical student career. First, try the less-daunting medical student journals. Reading, appraising and understanding journal articles is a skill that needs to be mastered; try to be proficient in this by the time you graduate.

Reading journals will teach you how to write a report or an article. Use the structure, referencing system and style of journal articles to guide you through your university work. Eventually you may submit your work to be published by your favourite journal.

Do not subscribe to the first journal you find. University libraries will usually have a good range of journals that you can access. Utilise these journals while researching for projects but also use this availability to look through journals you think may interest you before you pay the subscription. Look out for student discounts or discounts associated with organisation membership before paying the full subscription costs. *See* this website: www.freemedicaljournals.com.

Journal clubs

Find medical students with similar interests to you and set up a journal club. Each time the club meets up every member brings with them a published journal article and presents it for discussion. Journal clubs encourage critical analysis of articles, understanding and interest in reading journals.

> Before doing anything, ask yourself 'What is the point in me spending my time doing this?' 'Will it aid my learning or will a session in the library be more beneficial?' You know what you need to study better than any other individual . . . do not feel you must go to every timetabled clinic. Be wary of a review clinic . . . this will inevitably be of no educational benefit. If it is poor, ask to leave or make up an excuse . . . assess the teachers. Figure out who is good and who is bad. Use the good one until exhaustion. Always be proactive in seeking out the best learning opportunities. *(Ross Stewart, fourth-year medical student, Dundee)*

Making best use of time

Getting the right balance between private study and hands-on experience is difficult and different for every student. Tailor this balance to your learning needs, not just what is least effort or most exciting.

Prioritise your personal learning needs. For example, do not spend all day taking blood if you have never examined a patient's abdomen before. If you are finding activities on a clinical placement of no educational benefit, do something about it. Try and find an alternative area to work in or shadow a non-doctor healthcare professional.

Read up as you go. Make sure you have a copy of the *British National Formulary* (BNF) nearby so you can find out what all the drugs a patient is taking are for. Similarly, carry around reference ranges to help you interpret test results. A small reference book (e.g. the *Oxford Handbook of Clinical Medicine*) can be useful to quickly look up conditions you have not heard about. Regular reading up on topics you encounter will result in a slow but solid accumulation of knowledge.

> Ask questions. Being in a large group of people, a lot of whom you don't know is intimidating, but when something remains unclear to you it is highly likely that others in the group will be having the same problem. Through my own experience as a medical student, the knowledge I have gained from asking the experts about aspects I don't understand has been phenomenal and it tends to stay in the memory bank longer, too! It makes you look interested, stay interested and therefore helps you to learn. *(Esther Downham, third-year medical student, Dundee)*

Box 7.4 Tips for successful learning (Paul White, second-year medical student, St Andrews)

- *Do not try and learn it all at once – it's impossible!* The first time you learn something, aim to gain an overview. Each time you return to the topic (either through revision or in subsequent years of study) you should add a layer of knowledge on top of the last one. Repetition is the key: the more times you go over the same information the better you retain it.
- *Less is (sometimes) more* – there is a limit to how much you can take in. The less information you have to remember the easier it is. Overloading your brain (which is easily done in medicine) may jeopardise the retention of knowledge or information you already have. Be aware of your memory limits. Use mnemonics or other techniques to help to retain information – acting as a key to opening the door to more information locked away in your brain: you do not have to *actively* remember everything.
- *Strike a good balance* – a medical student is like no other student for the amount of work that has to be done! It is easy to do too much work. Make time for play as well as work. Too much work can result in burn-out. Spending two hours going out or playing sports allows your brain to relax enough to allow you to do more work later on. However, you need to find the right balance: too little work early on results in greater exam stress. If you build up vast amounts of unfinished work, it is very difficult to get back on top of things.
- *Learn appropriate study skills* – school is very different from university. You may realise that the techniques you used to learn and study in school may no longer be effective. Learning has to be quicker and with a lot more depth. Regularly evaluate your studying to identify areas for improvement. This does not necessarily mean putting in more hours, but thinking about how you can get the most out of the time you have. Repetitive reading, question cards and summary notes are a good use of studying time.
- *Learn information in a variety of ways* – read it, write it down, explain it to others, listen to it in lectures and answer questions: the more 'impressions' you have for the same piece of information the more likely you are to remember it.
- *Plan your day* – allocate time for study and play, and stick to it. It is easy to let things slip and procrastinate if you do not have set goals.
- *Know your limits* – you cannot know everything and you have to accept this; just always try your best.
- *Prepare for teaching* – reading about a topic before a formal teaching session will maximise the benefits of this learning experience.
- *Make it fun* – if you find it enjoyable you are more likely to retain information. Put difficult information into a story, make up funny phrases or use mnemonics.
- *Don't give up* – at times you are likely to get stressed and think about quitting. Everyone does. Just take one day at a time and try not to get bogged down with more work; you will look back at the end of the year and be grateful that you kept going. You may even say to yourself, 'Gaw, I actually know stuff!'

FURTHER READING

Abimbola S. Tips on buying textbooks. *StudentBMJ*. 2005; **13**: 335.

Patten D. What lies beneath: the use of three-dimensional projection in living anatomy teaching. *The Clinical Teacher*. 2007; **4**: 10-14.

Villaneuva T, Ravichandran B. Digesting journals. *StudentBMJ*. 2006; **14**: 266.

www.medicalmnemonics.com (A searchable site containing many mnemonics covering a wide range of specialties.)

CHAPTER 8

Exams

⫸ **Those that worry the most often have the least to worry about.**

Examinations are a major source of concern and anxiety. Unfortunately, they occur frequently in medical school. Medical schools throughout the UK have different teaching and assessment methods, each conforming to General Medical Council (GMC) guidelines. Various examination formats are required to assess medical students fully. Read on for the examination methods used in medical school and tips for success.

WHY DO EXAMS?

Exams are not always viewed as the best method of identifying potentially good doctors. However, they are the only way that is fair, relatively objective and regulated. To improve the quality, validity and fairness of examinations and assessments, medical schools should give you clear guidance on what is expected from you.

Exams should support the curriculum. Therefore medical exams are based upon course learning objectives. Medicine is a vast and diverse subject. Thus assessment methods must be varied and regular to provide good evidence that these objectives are being met.

Formative and summative exams

Exams are either *formative* or *summative*. You will probably undertake both types while at medical school so it is important that you understand the difference.

Formative exams are part of the learning process and do not count towards your degree. They produce useful feedback on your progress. You may be told whether you have 'passed' or 'failed' but are often not given the grades. Such examinations may be called 'mock' examinations. However, take them seriously because they can give an accurate impression of your ability. Good scores in formative exams can illustrate your potential should you encounter academic difficulties in the future.

Summative exams are those that count towards your degree or progress through the years.

GENERAL TIPS FOR SUCCESS IN ANY EXAM

Leave your mobile at home

It is astonishing how many people persist in taking their mobile phones into exams. It is incredibly stupid; being caught with a phone during an exam carries a high risk of failing that exam and facing disciplinary action from your university. Keep mobile phones and any other communication devices at home to make certain you are not accused of cheating.

Be timely

Know the venue of your exam and how to get there. Aim to reach the exam room at least half an hour early to allow for unforeseen hold-ups.

Read or listen to the question carefully

Be clear on what is being asked before you answer. In a practical exam do check if you are not sure. Many students, when asked to examine a patient, start to take a history. Similarly, if asked to examine the cardiovascular system, do not mention findings associated with the gastrointestinal system, especially if they are negative findings. Both errors waste time, make you appear unsure about what you are doing and invite difficult and irrelevant questions from the examiner.

Stop (breathe) and think before you answer

Exams do not usually require quick-fire questions and answers. You have time (as long as it takes to take a deep breath in and out) for contemplation, logical organisation and formulation of considered responses. Washing your hands in a practical exam demonstrates hygiene and provides a natural pause. Use this time wisely, do not panic and think about what you have been taught.

Plan your time

Calculate the number of questions you need to do per hour and how long you have for each question. For practical exams, time planning involves practising your techniques against the clock. Time warnings are often given in practical exams. Use these as a cue to sum-up what you have done or found out.

Do not use abbreviations

Abbreviations and acronyms can lead to confusion. Avoid these and demonstrate your knowledge by using full terms.

Find out what equipment you need

You often need a lab coat and stethoscope for practical exams. Other practical equipment is usually provided (e.g. pen torch, tourniquet or ophthalmoscope). For all exams consider taking a black pen, pencil, rubber and calculator (must not store text). Remember to use a see-through pencil case or plastic bag to carry your equipment to prevent false accusations of cheating.

Use all the information you are given

Examiners usually do not give you red herrings. Consider all the information you have been given and how it relates to the problem. You may have to think laterally, for example, not just the given conditions but the side effects of relevant treatment. Associations used in exams include: arthritis and long-term use of non-steroidal anti-inflammatory agents (e.g. ibuprofen) and asthma and steroid treatment. Stop and think before you dismiss any information.

Know the acceptable format for your answers

Some papers are computer-marked. For these you have to clearly write a letter, cross or line in a box that represents the answer you are giving. Make sure your answers are within the limits of the boxes otherwise your correct answer may be marked as wrong. Some institutions allow bullet points for short answer questions; this will save time, just make sure their use will not cause you to be marked down.

Know the marking system

Find out the marking scheme(s). For negative marking schemes, correct answers are given a positive value, blank or unanswered questions are marked as zero and wrong answers have a negative value. If your examinations are negatively marked, you will require a degree of confidence in order to submit an answer. This will depend on your self-confidence and the number of questions you have confidently answered already. If your paper is not negatively marked, attempt all questions. Some guesses, educated or not, may prove to be correct and boost your grades. Knowing the pass mark, or how it is worked out, will give you an idea of what you are aiming for.

First answer the questions you know

Answer the questions you are most confident about first to ensure that you have collected some points if you run out of time. Write provisional answers in pencil if you are unsure and fill them in with pen later once you have thought about them. Alternatively, you may be happier writing answers or notes on the question sheet first before transferring them to the answer sheet. Find a way that works for you. Just make sure you leave enough time to enter answers on the official sheet.

Leave time at the end for checking

Make sure that the answers you have given make sense and that you have included all the information that is requested of you.

TYPES OF EXAMINATION

> Schemes of assessment must take account of best practice, support the curriculum, make sure that the intended curricular outcomes are assessed and reward performance appropriately.[1]

Exams vary in the way you are examined, how the questions are asked and the subject areas you are being tested on. Indeed, there is also variation in the dates of exams. Early each year, ensure you know the examination methods you will be undergoing and when the examinations will be held. Do not assume the examination periods or techniques will be the same each year.

Short- and long-answer papers

Short-answer papers require you to write a few notes to answer or discuss a question or statement. For example, 'What are the risk factors for cervical cancer?' Some short-answer questions may comprise a step-by-step tour of the presentation, diagnosis, investigation and management of a particular condition.

Case-based exams follow the problem-based learning (PBL) (*see* Chapter 6) style of teaching. Case-based papers may be 'seen' or 'unseen'. Seen papers involve reading through a case and revising all the information relating to the 'learning objectives' prior to entering the exam. Thus, seen cases are primarily testing your knowledge. Unseen case-based exams are those in which a case is presented to you for the first time in the exam. You have to perform PBL steps such as cue identification, linking and hypothesis creation. Unseen cases are designed to test problem-solving, analytical and interpretation abilities.

Publication-based exams are set by some medical schools to assess comprehension, English writing and lay communication abilities. You have to read a passage of text, understand and interpret it, and then rephrase it in a coherent way, understandable to non-medically trained people.

Essay questions are pretty self-explanatory. You are given a title for an essay, or a number of essay titles from which you have to pick one, for example. Additional information on what you should include is sometimes provided. Essay questions have recently fallen out of favour because scoring involves an element of subjectivity and thus has potential for bias.[2]

Tips for success

Make copious relevant points. Only a prescribed number of marks are available for each specific point so do not write pages discussing only one thing. Equally, the more points you make, the more likely you are to cover all the items on the marking criteria.

Plan your answers. Essay-based questions require good, but rapid, planning at the beginning. Ensure you incorporate all the aspects they wish you to cover into your plan to prevent their omission if you rush at the end.

Spend the correct proportion of time answering each question based on the fraction of the total marks it represents.

Limited-answer papers

The presentation of such exams may vary; however, they generally include a question and a hidden answer. Papers such as these are employed widely across medical schools in all years. Questions may just be text or associated with 'slides', a picture or data. The format of the questions and answers can vary for different papers, as described below, and all may be associated with visual aids.

➡ *True and false questions* – statements for which you indicate whether they are true or false.

➡ *Multiple-choice questions (MCQs)* – a statement or question is followed by a number of answers. Mark each stem as correct/incorrect/do not know or the correct/incorrect stems, as instructed.

➡ *Extended matching questions (EMQs)* – a list of answers and a number of statements are given. You have to match the answers to the statements. You may be allowed to use the same answer more than once or more than one answer for each question.

Difficulties and frustrations can arise from these exams. You are unable to justify your answers, which is annoying if there are a number of right options and you have to choose 'the most appropriate' one. A lack of information is another common complaint. Lastly, you will often leave the exam with no idea how you have done and this can make the wait for the results tense.

Tips for success

How many answers are required? It is important to note whether you are supposed to be entering just one answer per question or all that are appropriate. If more than one answer is correct, but only one answer is required you should submit the most likely/common answer.

Is the correct answer the false or the true statement? Be alert to different questions on the same paper asking for the 'one correct' and the 'one false' answer.

Look for clues in the way the questions and answers are worded. General rules about the way in which questions or answers are worded can provide a clue to the correct response. For example, *never* and *always* often indicate false answers, as do exact statistical figures; things in medicine rarely occur this consistently. Similarly, vague words, such as *may*, *could* and *possibly*, often indicate a true statement.[3] Also beware of the use of negatives within a question: 'Which of these are *not* treatments of condition x?'

Think of the answer before looking at the choices. Sometimes looking at the choices can blur your thoughts. If your 'blind' answer is listed, it is likely to be correct.[4]

Exclude obvious wrong answers. Some questions may totally baffle you. Exclude all answers that are obviously wrong to increase the odds that you will guess the correct answer.

Believe in the quality of your revision. If you thought you knew the subject of the question well but have never heard of one of the answers, it is probably false.[3]

Practical exams

Practical exams often cause the most amount of anxiety because they involve one-on-one, face-to-face 'interrogation'. You cannot hide behind a pen and you feel foolish if you cannot answer or say something stupid.

Practical exams may be called:
➡ objective structured scientific examinations (OSSE)
➡ objective structured practical examinations (OSPEs)
➡ objective structured clinical examinations (OSCEs).

Practical exams usually consist of a string of 10–20 'stations' each lasting five to ten minutes. The content of each station depends on the module/year being tested. Each station is screened off and you are presented with scenarios, tasks, problems and/or clinical exercises (e.g. history-taking, physical examination, clinical or communication skills) to complete, solve or perform. For example, 'This patient has been complaining of blurred vision, please examine their vision'. At the end of the allotted time, you move on to the next station. 'Rest stations' that are empty stations are sometimes included; use this time to gather your thoughts and calm down before the next 'station'.

Senior medical students may undertake 'long cases' or objective structured long examination record (OSLER). These stations are 20–30 minutes in length. You are required to take a history and/or examine a patient and present the case (*see The Medical Student's Survival Guide 2: going clinical*). Finish by suggesting a management plan.

The objective nature of practical exams is maintained by use of standardised score sheets, from which each examiner works. The exams are structured to ensure continuity and fairness for each student. Consistency is ensured by the use of simulated patients or students in many cases. If real patients are used, allowances are made for the variation of symptoms and signs. Favoured in undergraduate and postgraduate settings, practical exams are designed to assess the required qualities for being a doctor (Figure 8.1), the most important of which are: safety in emergencies; competent history-taking; examination skills; basic clinical procedures; and, perhaps most importantly, professionalism.[5] Practical exams usually start with scenarios or questions that test basic knowledge. Questioning or requests gradually become more difficult to determine the extent of your knowledge. Questions will be asked until you do not know the answer; thus not knowing an answer does not mean you have failed. If you have answered questions for four of the allotted five minutes, you are likely to have passed that station.

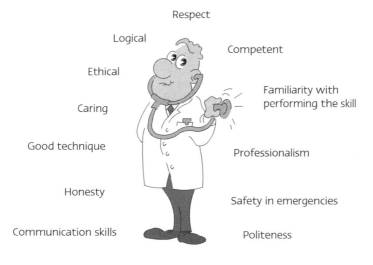

Respect

Logical

Competent

Ethical

Familiarity with
performing the skill

Caring

Good technique

Professionalism

Honesty

Safety in emergencies

Communication skills

Politeness

Figure 8.1 Qualities that practical exams are designed to test.

You may not find all the signs or reach a diagnosis and you may fail at least one station.[6] However, if you have shown yourself to be competent, safe and professional you will pass the exam.

Tips for success

Dress smartly. Demonstrate professionalism; do not turn up wearing trainers, jeans and a scruffy t-shirt. A suit may not be necessary, but you should be smart (no cartoon ties or logos). Be comfortable and respectable; do not find yourself kneeling on the floor doing basic life support in a restrictive shirt, mini-skirt and stilettos!

To speak or not to speak, what was the question? If it is not clear, check if the examiner wants you to perform a running commentary of your actions and findings while you are examining a patient; if not, perform one in your head in preparation for your presentation, which is sure to follow.

Demonstrate scrupulous personal hygiene. Make sure you have short clean nails, long hair is tied back and you do not smell of cigarettes and/or alcohol.

Smile as you enter the station. You may be nervous, feel like crying or hate the examiner; however, you will immediately put across a good impression if you enter with a warm and friendly smile. This will also appease and endear you to the simulated/real patients. A smile hides your nerves and makes you look confident under pressure.

Be confident. This is very difficult when you have a gross tremor and altered breathing. You also do not want to overcompensate and come across as arrogant or flippant. Aim to give the impression that you know what you are doing, have done it many times before, can cope under pressure and are competent in the particular task being examined. Use phrases such as, 'there is an expiratory wheeze' rather than 'I think there may be an expiratory wheeze'.

Wash your hands. For any task involving a procedure, examination, models, patients or simulated patients, ensure that you wash your hands. At the beginning of the station use the alcohol rub or gel provided, or state that you wish to wash your hands. Do not forget to do the same at the end. Some medical schools score a point just for doing this. Hygiene is incredibly important in general clinical practice so make a habit of it.

Introduce yourself and gain consent. Points are often awarded just for adequately doing this. Make sure you practise it; rolling your full name (not nicknames or informal versions), position, reason for doing what you want to do and information required for consent off your tongue is much easier if you have done it many times before.

Structure your response and be systematic. You know the generic approaches to history-taking, examination (e.g. inspection, palpation, percussion and auscultation) and presentation of patients (*see The Medical Student's Survival Guide 2: going clinical*) so use them! Time pressure, stress and anxiety make many students completely abandon these templates and completely miss out large sections of tasks they would easily perform otherwise. This is frustrating for the student and examiner who both know that the underlying knowledge and ability is there.

Look at the equipment provided. The available equipment is usually relevant and there to be used. Glance at the equipment table at the start of the exam to help you structure your actions. If there is time to spare at the end, have another look at the equipment and think of the uses of any untouched objects.

Do not hurt or embarrass the patient. Doing either of these things may, quite rightly, result in immediate failure. Check for pain before starting an examination and ask the patient to inform you if they feel 'discomfort'. Do not maul the patient like a ball of dough. Gentleness is also required if you have to break bad news or talk about sensitive issues. You will fail if you upset the patient by being abrupt and/or inappropriate. Ensure the patient is covered/dressed before you finish, they may require assistance.

If you really do not know the answer, say 'I don't know'. You will not waste time and you may even be given a hint in order to move the questions on, perhaps to something you do know.

Listen to the examiner. If an examiner appears to be steering you down another path to the one you have commenced, go with them. They are usually trying to help. For example, 'Are you sure that is the correct syringe?' probably means 'That is not the correct syringe, find another one'. You will not endear yourself to an examiner if you demonstrate incompetence or a lack of knowledge and then ignore useful advice.

Find out if there are any 'killer stations'. 'Killer stations' are those that, if failed, cause you to fail your entire examination. Although more common in postgraduate exams, they may be present at your medical school. Find out which skills or knowledge are tested in killer stations. Then, make sure you know any potential 'killer stations' like the back of your hand.

Oral examinations

Oral examinations (viva) are often used to categorise those at the extremes of the exam achievement spectrum. For example, if you only just failed an exam, a successful performance in a viva may result in an overall pass. At the other end of the spectrum, if your work has been of very high quality you may be given a viva to gain a distinction grade. Oral examinations are also used to assess the extent to which a good project is the student's own work.

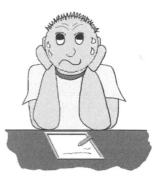

Oral examinations are delivered by varying numbers of professionals, from each of whom you will receive questions. Oral examinations often require a vast depth and breadth of knowledge.

REVISION

⑊➡   **Find a penny and pick it up and all day long you will have a penny . . . do not just rely on luck.**

Key areas of knowledge that often arise in exams are found in Box 8.1, and tips for successful revision may be found in Box 8.2.

Learn and prepare through a solid, basic understanding

Learn from a basic level. This allows you to work out some answers rather than just recalling lists of bare facts. Find out how something happens, not just that it does.

Prepare well in advance

Medicine is a vast, broad and in-depth subject. You cannot cram for medical school exams and you cannot rely on luck. There is no way you will learn everything you need to know at the last minute; work thoroughly and consistently throughout medical school. Take every learning opportunity you can. The anecdote your consultant told you during a quiet clinic may be an answer to a future exam question. Some medical schools do their final exams in the fourth year of a five-year course; find out when your finals will be during your first year. It could result in a significant difference in pre-finals learning time.

All the exams you take are based upon your curriculum learning objectives; thus, go through these early in your revision. Ideally, you should refer to these throughout the relevant modules to ensure you are learning everything the first time round.

Plan your revision

Making a revision plan is the most commonly used avoidance technique for revision. It suddenly seems crucial that a neatly coloured-in plan is present before revision can take place. However, revision plans can be very useful, just be realistic and task-based. Plan the topics you want to cover in a day or week, rather than the amount of time you are going to spend revising. This will allow for good days and bad days, and will also mean that you do not spend a whole two-hour revision slot getting bogged down with unnecessary minutiae.

Make your plan well in advance (months/weeks rather than days). There is so much to cover that you will not do it all in a week. Also, if you discover a topic you need to go back to there will be plenty of time to do so.

Get your hands on as many past papers as you (legally) can

Working through past papers from your university will demonstrate the format and types of questions you will be faced with. Get your hands on all the past papers your university releases; practice makes perfect. Be disciplined and undertake 'mocks' in which you independently write the paper to time. Afterwards, you can mark your mock paper by looking up answers, even the ones you are almost certain about, in textbooks. Discuss your answers with your peers; you can help each other to understand the paper.

Box 8.1 Key areas to know about

- Appropriate use and interpretation of history, examination, investigation and planning of management
- History-taking and differentials of common relevant conditions
- Examination of relevant body systems
- Ethical issues – autonomy, beneficience (do good), consent and confidentiality, do no harm, justice and equity
- Professionalism – treat the patient (and the exam) with respect
- Basic life support (BLS) and/or advance life support (ALS)
- Appropriate medical emergencies – recognition and management, for example acute severe asthma, arrhythmias, myocardial infarction, diabetic ketoacidosis, hypoglycaemia, left ventricular failure

---

Find out previous topics

It is much easier to guess possible questions in short- and long-answer papers than it is for limited-answer papers. However, studying past papers and revision books will give you an impression of the common topics in medical school exams.

Reflect on previous experiences

Only you know your exam weaknesses. Do you always fail to finish on time? If so have plenty of practice doing timed past papers. Is a lack of correct knowledge or understanding the problem? Look at the questions you are asked by your university and practise as many similar questions as possible. Ask your tutors' advice on the breadth and depth of knowledge you will require for each exam.

Box 8.2 Tips for successful revision (Paul White, second-year medical student, St Andrews)

- Less is (sometimes) more – cramming too much information can cause you to lose knowledge already stored
- Be organised and plan ahead
- Make it fun and keep it interesting
- Stay disciplined – try to keep to a study plan
- Read, memorise, reflect, understand and recite
- Do practice questions and papers to build up confidence
- Continually re-evaluate your working style and change it if it is not efficient
- Have regular breaks – give your brain chance to relax
- Do not copy textbooks – it is better just to use textbooks for reference

---

Do you want a revision partner?

Consider revising with friends. However, choose your companions wisely; too much messing about will waste time and too much arrogance may reduce your confidence. Much can be learned when several heads tackle questions and scenarios. Some people are more focused when working with others because it is harder to act on distractions when you are in company. Teach each other, test theories between yourselves and provide constructive criticism on practical skills.

> My friends and I commandeered a project room over the May holiday weekend and put the paediatric milestones on a whiteboard, so they were there all weekend as we covered other revision topics. We played a 'milestone game' over the weekend with three people: one tells another what age to act; the 'actor' has to remember what the appropriate milestones were for that age and act it out; and the third person examines the 'baby' and works out from the behaviour what age it is. This was absolutely hilarious in addition to being a really useful study tool, and it certainly lightened the day a bit in between psychiatry, suicide assessments and reading chest X-rays. (Scott, fifth-year medical student, Glasgow)

Books

Revision books are so numerous it is impossible to list them all. However, there are a number of different types of revision books that you should be aware of so you choose those that best suit your revision style and your university's exam format.

➡ Lists of questions with the correct answers given but no explanation.

➡ Questions with detailed answers (e.g. the One Stop Doc series, *Ten Teachers' Self Assessment in Gynaecology and Obstetrics*[7]).

➡ Notes on the subject (Lecture Notes series, Oxford Handbook series).

➡ Notes on the subject with revision questions (Crash Course series, *Pass Finals*,[8] Master Medicine/Surgery series).

➡ Revision books associated with specific text books (*Ten Teachers' Self Assessment in Gynaecology and Obstetrics*,[7] *Illustrated Self Assessment in Paediatrics*,[9] MCQs in *Clinical Medicine*,[10] *Pass Finals*[8]).

Courses

Useful local or university-based revision courses exist but change regularly and are often arranged at short notice. For more information about these, ask your tutors. National revision courses are usually sponsored by professional organisations, usually carry an attendance fee and are commonly aimed at students taking their final examinations. The format of these national courses is usually similar year to year.

> I chose to go on the Medicine and Surgery revision courses (*see* www.askdoctorclarke.com) that were held seven weeks before my final exams. I was apprehensive in case it increased my anxiety. However, I thoroughly enjoyed it. The pre-course work gave an idea of the depth of knowledge required. The course itself consisted of two long days, but I felt like I learnt more than I would ever learn on my own. Bob taught us mnemonics, examination techniques and even a dance to help us to remember information! It was not intimidating as we were not forced to practise examinations in front of everyone; however, we were encouraged to practise sequences we had just been shown with a partner sitting next to us. Knowledge and tips were supported by the comprehensive course booklets, which also contained past-course notes to read through in our own time. (*Lizzie, fifth-year medical student, Manchester*)
>
> As for the course (www.askdoctorclarke.com), it was the first time in ages I felt I was actually being 'taught'; problem-based learning is all very well, but it's nice to have some guidance once in a while. Overall, I thought it was excellent, really well oriented towards the clinical examination. (*Susan, fourth-year medical student, Liverpool*)

Revision courses are not without criticism but such negative attitudes may be a reflection of the different revision styles among medical students. Some prefer to work at their own pace, in small groups or with individual tutors. For those who are interested, revision courses can be money well spent.

The general purpose of revision courses is to focus students on the knowledge and skills required to pass their examinations. They are not designed to coach students to reach honours level. A good revision course will highlight common exam topics (which do not always correlate with common diseases) and help you to refine your clinical skills.

National revision courses usually tour around the UK so you often have a choice of time and place. By definition, they are *revision* courses so do not use them as an introduction to a topic or you will not keep up. The pace of progression from topic to topic is rapid.

Organisations will advertise their revision courses by saying that people who attend generally do better in their exams. This has to be taken with a pinch of salt. It may be purely that those students who have the motivation and enthusiasm to attend revision courses are those more likely to pass anyway. However, this should not put you off. Even if you know most of the content of a revision course you may pick up tips and advice for refining your skills and knowledge. It may also serve as a comfort blanket when you realise you know more than you thought you did.

> Thanks for such a great weekend. I was a bit dubious about revision courses, and people had said things like 'Oh, it's just for people who haven't done any revision', but I found it really useful. It was a good opportunity to test myself in a non-threatening environment, and as I actually haven't done much revision 'Surgery for Finals' (www. askdoctorclarke.com) has served as a good basis in case I don't get round to doing any more! *(Rosie, fifth-year medical student, Manchester)*
>
> I felt that the hernia and varicose veins examinations went really well for me, and this was thanks to your revision course (www.askdoctorclarke. com). I felt confident in what I was saying to the examiners, and got the impression that they could tell I knew what I was talking about. I have never done a vascular surgery placement during my training, and my only general surgery placement was in upper gastrointestinal surgery, so I hadn't seen a great many hernias in my time! I would have really struggled in those stations had I not attended your revision course. *(Sam, fifth-year medical student, Manchester)*

Professional Medical Education

Professional Medical Education (PME) runs a series of courses that help students consolidate the knowledge that they acquire throughout medical school. Difficult subjects are made easy and simple to understand. Look at the PME website (www. freefees.co.uk) for comments they have received from attendees of previous courses.

Courses for first year students cover anatomy. The courses also cater for year three OSCEs and revision for finals. All course lecturers are experts in their field.

Dr Bob Clarke's 'Medicine for Finals' and 'Surgery for Finals'

Dr Bob Clarke has been helping students pass their exams for more than 20 years. His one-day courses 'Medicine for Finals' and 'Surgery for Finals' are sponsored by the British Medical Association (BMA) and held at hospitals and universities throughout the UK. These highly acclaimed courses provide a comprehensive approach to common exam questions, with an emphasis on clinical skills and plenty of opportunities to ask questions. Illustrated booklets are provided with each course to supplement the information given, which many students find invaluable for structuring their revision; it is useful to annotate these with the anecdotes and techniques discussed during the day. For more information on dates, venues, previous attendees' comments and course content, visit the Ask Doctor Clarke website (www.askdoctorclarke.com).

Medical Defence Union revision courses

Medical Defence Union (MDU) revision courses are held up and down mainland UK between February and April. The MDU courses include surgery finals, medicine finals, pediatrics finals and third-year objective structured clinical examination (OSCE) revision. The MDU offers discounts to members signed up for their Foundation 1 year for the finals courses. The MDU medicine and surgery courses are each two days. For more information on their revision courses, visit the MDU website (www.the-mdu.com).

Medical Protection Society finals revision courses

The Medical Protection Society sponsors finals revision courses for students. They are two-day courses that start with a pre-course MCQ and EMQ paper. The medicine course contains revision tips for the cardiovascular, respiratory, gastrointestinal, endocrine and neurological systems, as well as rheumatology, haematology and renal. The surgical day covers the hip, knee, shoulder, hand, spine, lumps and bumps, breast, vascular system and abdomen. Both days cover relevant emergencies and have 'clinics' during which you can ask the presenters questions. A fee is payable (£100 in 2007), but many attendees of such courses think it well worth it.

   The courses are run across England, Scotland and Ireland. For more information on costs, venues, dates and previous students' comments, visit the website (www.medicalprotection.org/medical/united_kingdom/students/revision_courses).

Websites
Doctors.net.uk

Free registration with Doctors.net.uk is very worthwhile. There are various features on the website (www.doctors.net.uk) but one of the most useful for revision is the 'education' area that contains tutorials. Questions guide you through tutorials covering diagnosis and management of some important conditions. Doctors.net. uk contains information on a number of relevant articles, diagrams and guidelines. The site also has a specific revision section, including practice OSCEs and X-ray quizzes, crib sheets providing the key points of exam knowledge and sources of entertainment for revision breaks.

Ask Doctor Clarke

The Ask Doctor Clarke website (www.askdoctorclarke.com) provides useful documents and videos detailing important conditions and techniques of clinical examination. Dr Clarke's website complements his national series of revision courses. He encourages email feedback from students about their exams and updates his website and revision courses accordingly. Information from the website provides a good base for further revision. Registration is free for UK clinical students.

> The Ask Doctor Clarke website (www.askdoctorclarke.com) is FANTASTIC – especially the videos – which I used a lot. What a brilliant idea. (*Emma, fifth-year medical student, St George's*)
>
> I found it extremely useful, and my housemates and I watched all the examination videos on the website (www.askdoctorclarke.com) before the OSCE. (*Shamira, fifth-year medical student, Southampton*)

One examination.com

One examination.com (www.oneexamination.com) is an interactive web-based revision course. There is a subscription charge to access the site on a four-monthly basis (discounts are available for MDU members). Try the interactive MCQs, SAQs and EMQs, and compare your results with other subscribers. After each question you receive a score and most provide an explanation of the answer. Your scores are interpreted in order to illustrate your weaker areas, allowing you to focus your revision on these. The website contains book reviews, a journal in which you can log your thoughts, plans and feelings about your revision and a section containing the latest medical news to ensure you are up to date on the 'hot topics'.

Medicalfinals.co.uk

Medicalfinals.co.uk (www.medicalfinals.co.uk) is a website designed for medical students approaching their final examinations, although most of the content is useful for all medical students. Through the site you can book to attend mock OSCEs held in Belfast, as well as accessing MCQs, tutorials, image resources, exam advice and online OSCEs. The website offers links to revision courses and other useful organisations.

YORACLE

YORACLE (Your Online Revision And Clinical Learning Environment) was devised by two Leicester medical students. The website (www.yoracle.com) encourages other medical students to share their revision material online. Content of the site is peer-reviewed and graded. Free registration is required to access the site. YORACLE contains revision notes, book reviews, case studies, elective advice and activities to do during your revision breaks.

Fleshandbones

The Fleshandbones website (www.fleshandbones.com) is a free learning resource for medical students, and contains a 'revision centre'. Interactive MCQ-style revision questions are marked straight after your attempt, by a negative marking system, so you immediately see your score and, in many cases, an explanation as to why the answer is so. The revision centre also provides links to OSCE revision material, mnemonics and tips from other students on getting through your exams. There is a section called 'survival guides' that has condensed 'need-to-know' information into revision notes; useful for a quick run-through to check you have not missed any vital topics. Finally, the revision centre has a section that lists, with a short paragraph on each, the 100 most important topics as judged by the editor of the Crash Course series of revision books along with a focus group of junior doctors at the Kent and Canterbury Hospital and the East Kent GP Vocational Training Scheme.

Surgical tutor

The surgical tutor website (www.surgical-tutor.org.uk) has a free and complete 'revision package' for medical students. Although the MCQ questions are not as extensive as some other sites, the answers are explained. There are tutorials on a vast number of surgical-related topics as well as resources for the surgical enthusiast, such as details of and quotes from past and influential surgeons. Impressive radiology and pathology galleries provide a variety of images that are each accompanied by a paragraph explaining the important features and diagnosis.

Clinicaltutor

The clinicaltutor website (www.clinicaltutor.com) contains a vast array of revision questions. You can use the site to 'build your own paper' by choosing your level of study, how many questions you want and the topics for your questions. You complete the paper under timed conditions before it is negatively marked. Full explanations of the answers are available.

Internet Pathology Laboratory for Medical Education

If it is pathology you need to revise, the Internet Pathology Laboratory for Medical Education of the Florida State University College of Medicine (http://medlib.med.utah.edu/WebPath/EXAM/EXAMIDX.html) provides a good number of slide-based MCQ questions. The questions are subdivided into the different systems of the body. You have to select the answers you believe to be correct and a response to that answer will be displayed.

Neurologic exam

The Neurologic exam website (http://library.med.utah.edu/neurologicexam/html/home_exam.html) provides tutorials and quizzes on the major neurological topics. It provides information and videos on the anatomy, a normal examination and the findings of an abnormal examination for each topic. Interactive MCQs are available and contain explanations for the answers. Although the site does not contain a vast array of information, it covers the main areas you will need as an undergraduate.

NeuroNet

NeuroNet (http://umed.med.utah.edu/neuronet) provides tutorials and quizzes on a number of clinical neurological topics. The interactive MCQs provide responses and marks immediately after each question. The site also contains cases with accompanying short-answer questions. Although the cases are designed for small group work and do not include answers, they may be a good basis for your revision if you use other resources to check your responses.

Keeping sane while revising

Revision periods are tough so look after yourself. Medical student exams are not your first exams; you have done well in the past to be where you are. Think about the strategies you used in the past and re-use those that were effective

Commonly heard by medical students is the phrase 'they want to pass you'. Some take this quite literally and enter the exams believing that passing is their right. Others gain no reassurance from this and will only be calmed upon receipt of a pass mark. The phrase is pretty accurate providing you have worked adequately during your time at medical school and are safe and courteous during the exam.

Maintain useful friendships. Some friends are more helpful to work with and others are better to relax with; choose friends appropriately for each situation. You can always return to your usual social routines after the exams.

Avoid unhelpful acquaintances. Do not spend time with people who wind up you and the rest of the medical student population by loudly stating the minutiae of everything at any available moment. They are only talking about what they know to avoid what they do not – pay no attention.

Take guilt-free breaks. Regularly do anything that takes you away from books, computers and notes. Go for a walk, go shopping or watch a bit of television. Do not feel guilty for taking time out, you need it.

Listen to your body. Stop studying if it is just 'not going in'. Your body is telling you that you need a break. When you have had a rest, a break or the morning/

afternoon off, you will be surprised how easy work then becomes. You are achieving nothing by staring at text, thinking about how little you are learning. Start revising early to provide leeway to have bad revision days.

Keep healthy. Get plenty of sleep, eat healthily and do not overdo the caffeine or alcohol.

Listen to Mozart. Listening to Mozart has been associated with better learning in college students – if all else fails, give it a go!

ASSESSMENTS AND EVALUATIONS

Assessments and evaluations are completed throughout medical school. The functions of such assessments may be to:

➡ determine your fitness to practice as a junior doctor
➡ ensure that your medical course is of high quality
➡ record your application and motivation to your work
➡ assess your computer and communication skills.

Your fitness to practice is evaluated by assessing your qualities in relation to depth and breadth of knowledge, skills, professional attitudes and behaviour.[1] The healthcare professionals who supervise you may be required to complete such evaluations. In addition, you will have to evaluate your own progress.

You are required to fill out assessment forms that evaluate the course, provided by the university. For these to be effective you need to be honest about what you think worked well and what you think needs to be changed.

THE FUTURE

There has been evidence that the different assessment processes between all medical schools has resulted in varying standards among graduates. Indeed, there is also a difference in the preparedness of graduates for their work as a junior doctor between medical schools. Therefore a national licensing process is under consideration; such as those within the USA and Canada. Keep up to date with progress in this area.[11] See the GMC website (www.gmc-uk.org) and the BMA website (www.bma.org).

The Universities Medical Assessment Partnership (UMAP) is a project that started in 2003 and is working towards building a common bank of written exam assessments for undergraduate medicine across the UK. UMAP has been formed to create a means by which inter-medical school core knowledge attainments can be compared. Each medical school involved in UMAP holds workshops with their own staff to write and submit questions in a prescribed format. UMAP is good news for you, as exam questions may become more evidence based and better formulated. Practice questions are available on the website (www.umap.org.uk). GOOD LUCK!

FURTHER READING

Bickle I. Mastering EMQs. *StudentBMJ*. 2002; **10**: 402.

Cantillon P. Mastering exam technique. *StudentBMJ*. 2000; **8**: 363–5.

Malik S. Many heads make light work of med school exams. *StudentBMJ*. 2006; **14**: 256–7.

CHAPTER 9

Projects

Written projects often comprise the end of a student-selected component (SSC) (*see* Chapter 15). Projects may also be required for the core components of your course. So how can you make sure your work is up to scratch?

> The practice of medicine is distinguished by the need for judgement in the face of uncertainty. Doctors take responsibility for these judgements and their consequences. A doctor's up-to-date knowledge and skills provide the basis for such judgements because so much of medicine's unpredictability calls for wisdom as well as technical ability. Doctors must be clearer about what they do and how and why they do it.[1]

Projects teach required skills, such as:
➡ evaluating effectiveness against evidence
➡ development and use of research skills
➡ analysis and use of numerical data.

When formulating objectives at the start of a project, try to tailor them to fulfil these skills.

EVIDENCE-BASED MEDICINE

Evidence-based medicine (EBM) is the buzz-phrase of current medical practice. A decision-making process based on available high-quality evidence, EBM is used in all specialties and fields of medicine. All healthcare professionals are encouraged to practise EBM. Therefore, the projects you undertake in medical school will assess your working knowledge of EBM.

EBM demonstrates population, rather than individual, medicine. Critical appraisal of the quality of available evidence is thus required to calculate risk and effectiveness (in terms of health and cost) of practices, procedures and treatments for each individual patient.

EBM is too huge to be described here. During your undergraduate training, learn how:

➡ to read and critically evaluate research papers
➡ research can be applied to clinical practice.

Some medical schools run EBM courses, attend these if possible. Start your journey into EBM by reading 'Evidence-based medicine: what it is and what it isn't'[2] and *How to Read a Paper: the basics of evidence based medicine.*[3]

If you develop an interest in EBM the *Evidence Based Medicine* journal (http://ebm.bmjjournals.com) provides information on performing research as well as publishing recent research findings.

Useful websites[4]

➡ The Centre for Evidence Based Medicine at the University of Oxford has designed a website (www.cebm.net) to assist professionals at any stage of familiarity with EBM. It explains what EBM is, how to practise it and how to teach it to others. It also contains a 'toolbox' to assist you in making EBM-related calculations, setting focused clinical questions and understanding relevant terms.
➡ The Centre for Health Evidence, based at the University of Alberta, has designed a useful website (www.cche.net) that contains users' guides for EBM (originally published in the *Journal of the American Medical Association*).
➡ The University of Toronto's Centre for Evidence Based Medicine has a website (www.cebm.utoronto.ca) offering tools that can help you understand EBM and its processes. The website also serves as support for the book *Evidence-based Medicine: how to practice and teach EBM.*[5]
➡ The Bandolier learning zone contains links to information to assist self-directed learning on EBM. The website (www.jr2.ox.ac.uk/bandolier/learnzone.html) covers understanding trials and meta-analysis, calculations, guidelines and health economics.

RESEARCH

⫸ **What should we be doing and how should we do it?**

You need to develop an understanding of existing and new research. You may undertake your own research while at medical school. Therefore, learn how to design and evaluate useful research. Although not covered in depth here, plenty of information is easily available.

Gather information on your topic to:

➡ establish whether your proposed research has already been performed

➡ predict the likely outcome of your research
➡ act as a foundation for your research.

Details of previous research can be found using a literature search (*see below*) and websites providing evaluations of past research (*see* 'Evaluating articles', p. 107).

Participants of research must be allocated to different conditions. Learn the techniques for doing this. For example, randomisation ensures each participant has an equal chance of entering any of the research conditions.

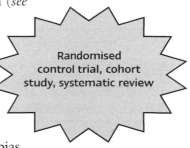

Randomised control trial, cohort study, systematic review

Understand sources of bias in research and how these can be reduced or eliminated. Think about how bias may arise from/through:
➡ recruitment of participants
➡ participant responses
➡ treatment of the participants by the researcher/doctor
➡ publication
➡ unaccounted-for variables.

Research can be divided into two categories: therapeutic and non-therapeutic research. Although this distinction is increasingly blurred, it describes the difference between research that involves personal benefit to the participant (therapeutic) and research that does not (non-therapeutic).

To get you started on any research, first consider four main aspects of its design:[6]
➡ the subjects or group(s) of subjects to be studied
➡ intervention that will be tested
➡ what comparison will be made – to subjects, group, alternative intervention
➡ outcome(s) of interest.

Research ethics committees

The Local Research Ethics Committee (LREC) or a Multicentre Research Ethics Committee (MREC) must approve all research. The Central Office for Research Ethics Committees (COREC) (www.corec.org.uk) co-ordinates the LRECs and MRECs in England, Scotland, Northern Ireland and Wales.

In order to gain ethical approval you must detail every aspect of your proposed research on two forms; the NHS Research Ethics Committee (REC) Application Form and the NHS Research and Development (R&D) Application Form. Your medical school must first approve any research you undertake as a student and you must have a supervisor. Medical schools have a dedicated ethics approval process for medical student research projects.

Applications can take time to go through the ethics committees. If any amendments have to be made, your research design will need updating before resubmitting the application. Thus, complete the application forms as early as you possibly can.

AUDIT

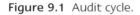 **What are we doing? Are we doing what we should be doing? How can we change what we are doing to make it better?**

Participate in audits as soon as possible. Many medical students have experience of audit by the time they graduate, which can be valuable on job application forms. Audit involves assessing clinical performance against standards set out in healthcare.

Be clear about how audit differs from research. Audit involves comparing what is happening against what should be happening in order to improve patient care and/or service provision. Research involves the acquisition of new knowledge and information.

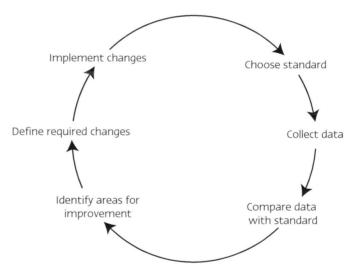

Figure 9.1 Audit cycle.

Audit involves a number of clearly defined steps, usually described in a cycle (Figure 9.1). The first involves defining the variable(s) to be audited. An appropriate standard, against which the variable will be assessed, should be chosen based on widely used guidelines and best practice. Next is the data-collection phase. This can be time-consuming, depending on the quantity and type of data being collected. Data collection can occur *retrospectively* (i.e. data from past events) or *prospectively* (i.e. data is collected as it happens). Once all data are collected they are compared with the previously identified standard and any areas for improvements are identified. Changes and those who should implement them must be defined following detection of deficits in performance. Once the new changes have been implemented for an adequate period of time the audit is repeated.

Audit should be led by a professional involved in the area of clinical activity under review; however, as a medical student you can collect and interpret data. You are expected to undertake audit regularly once you graduate.

Clinical governance

Clinical governance is: 'A framework through which NHS organisations are accountable for continually improving the quality of their services and safeguarding high standards of care by creating an environment in which excellence in clinical care will flourish'.[6]

You are likely to hear the term 'clinical governance' throughout your clinical placements, but do you know what it means? Clinical governance is related to audit and is the mechanism by which standards in healthcare are maintained. It works on the basis that individuals should be accountable for setting, maintaining and monitoring standards of performance in achieving high quality clinical care. This may involve inviting individuals and groups of healthcare workers to identify and implement best practice. Clinical governance maintains standards by ensuring that:[7]

➡ fully functioning systems are in place to monitor the quality of clinical practice
➡ clinical practice is reviewed and improved (using clinical audit and risk management strategies)
➡ clinical practitioners adhere to and practise by the standards set by national professional regulatory bodies; this is performed through effective management of poorly performing colleagues, continuing education and encouragement of evidence-based clinical practice.

Projects you undertake at medical school will teach you skills that ensure you can practice EBM and understand the processes of clinical governance, *see* the website www.cgsupport.nhs.uk.

Guidelines and standards

Guidelines and standards are developed locally and nationally. They are evidence-based and devised under consultation with relevant healthcare professionals. Therefore, they outline best practice and should be followed or met when appropriate.

Standards of care are often laid down in national service frameworks (NSFs). NSFs set out the requirements of a healthcare service, how services should be delivered and a timescale within which changes should occur. Similar to guidelines, standards are developed in consultation with health professionals, service users, managers and other external healthcare or patient agencies.

Sources of guidelines and standards include:

➥ Prodigy (www.prodigy.nhs.uk)
➥ National Institute for Clinical Excellence (NICE) (www.nice.org.uk)
➥ www.nelh.nhs.uk/guidelinesfinder/
➥ SIGN (www.sign.ac.uk/index.html)
➥ NSFs (www.nelh.nhs.uk/nsf/default.htm).

STATISTICS

Whether you are undertaking research or trying to understand published research, you need to understand statistics. For example, drug companies often make claims that sound too good to be true – statistics knowledge will help you to determine if they are.

A full description and explanation of the statistics you require as a medical student is beyond the scope of this book. However, you will be introduced to the level and type of understanding you will require.

Learn the different ways data can be collected in order to establish the correct statistical tests to analyse it. Data may be:

➥ *Nominal* (mutually exclusive groups) – for example, whether a person is male or female
➥ *Ordinal* (ranked exclusive groups) – for example, breathlessness scored on the New York Heart Association Classification
➥ *Continuous* (values that occur anywhere along a continuum) – for example, height/weight.

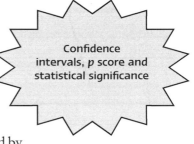

Confidence intervals, *p* score and statistical significance

An overall impression of a set of data may be represented by an average value. An average value can be calculated as the:

➥ *mean* (all values added together and divided by the number of values summated)
➥ *mode* (value occurring most frequently)
➥ *median* (middle value when all values are ordered from smallest to largest).

Understand the difference between each and when expression of one is more appropriate than the others. Average values do not always accurately demonstrate data; sometimes the spread of data is also required. This is expressed as the *variance* (spread of values either side of a mean), *standard deviation* (range of values within which a certain proportion of the sample will lie) and *standard error* (the range within which the population mean will lie as calculated from the sample mean).

Many data in medicine fit a 'normal' (Gaussian or bell-shaped) distribution. It is essential you familiarise yourself with the normal distribution and the fact that with this distribution of values the mean, median and mode average values are equal to each other.

Comparative statistics refers to comparing two groups of data. Concepts to grasp include the definitions of *hypothesis* and *null hypothesis*; simply, these are the questions being tested by the research. Statistical tests are used to identify differences between two groups of data and, if present, whether the differences are significant. The appropriate test depends upon whether the data fit a normal distribution and the types of data being examined. The significance of any differences is given along with a *confidence interval*; a range of values within which the true mean will lie in the specified percentage of cases.

Correlation is used to investigate the relationship between two variables. Variables may be *directly related* (one goes up and so does another), *inversely related* (one goes up and the other goes down) or *not related*.

The benefit or harm of one treatment against another may be recorded in terms of the *relative risk*; the change in the probability of an event occurring in a group in which the treatment is given compared to a group which did not receive that treatment. If the relative risk is 1, this means the risk of an event occurring in each group is equal. Develop an appreciation of the differences between relative and absolute risk.

Number needed to treat

There is a lot to learn regarding statistics. For a successful and informed degree and career in medicine you will need to understand all the items introduced above. However, the interpretation of results may be simplified for beginners by making sure you can answer the following three questions, every time you have to perform data analysis:[8]

➡ What is the direction of the result?
➡ What is the size of the effect?
➡ What is the statistical significance of the result?

LITERATURE SEARCHES

If you need to research a topic you should perform a literature search. Without knowing how to perform literature searches you cannot practise EBM; research and guidance will not magically appear before you. A literature search is the process by which you find published articles related to the topic you are interested in.

What are you looking for?

Decide what information you want to search for. Be as specific as possible. So much information is available you must sieve out irrelevant material as early as possible. Ask yourself the following questions and use your answers to help you decide which words to use for your literature search.

➡ To which group of individuals, conditions or problems does your project apply? (For example, the elderly.)

➡ Which interventions, treatments or conditions do you want information on? (For example, heart attack, myocardial infarction.)

➡ Do you want to compare one intervention, treatment or condition with another? If so, what are you going to use in this comparison? (For example, stroke, cerebrovascular accident.)

➡ What are the outcomes that you are interested in? (For example, death, mortality.)

Can other phrases, words or terms be substituted for the answers you have given? If so, write down all the alternatives, as illustrated in the bullet points. The final answers are your 'keywords' that you will input to conduct your literature search.

Where should you look?

There are many electronic databases of medicine and health-related research, through which you can search for relevant literature. Information is obtained via search mechanisms, into which you type your keywords. This results in a list of matching articles.

> Refine your search further by combining two
> searches using different relevant terms

Medical students can access electronic databases through university library web pages, via the National Electronic Library of Health (NELH) or through home computers. Useful databases include general medical databases such as Medline and Embase, and specialty-specific databases such as PsycINFO.

Each database is slightly different, but all have instructions. Find the search page and enter your keywords. The most specific searches are for documents that include all your keywords. If no articles match your keywords, redo the search using broader keywords. For example, change a specific name to a class of drug. If you

> Find the limit or filter function in the database to allow you to select
> specific types of document, e.g. one type of research, one language

have combined keywords, search for each one separately to see if this results in any matching documents. You can always combine two searches at a later stage.

If you have performed your search and thousands of articles have been matched, attempt to refine your search in order to only match those with direct relevance. Try using more keywords or combine a couple of searches you have performed, or use more specific terms.

Accessing the articles highlighted by the literature search

All articles matching your keywords will be listed. Usually you are given the option to print, save or email this list. Information within the list includes the author's name, title of the article and details of publication (usually a journal). Sometimes direct links take you to electronic versions of the article.

Your university website may have links to electronic journals. Search for the journal(s) you require and follow the appropriate link(s). Alternatively, your university library may hold a number of backdated paper journals that you can search manually.

You can ask library staff to order a copy of the article for you. There is often a charge associated with this. Ask your university librarians for more details.

Visit the journal homepage directly. Journal homepages have an archive link and a search function. Input the details of the article you want or follow the appropriate links in the archive to find your article. If you still cannot access an article, you will have to either email the corresponding author of the article and/or pay for a copy; details will be found on the journal site.

Athens

Access to full text versions of articles often requires a subscription. However, subscriptions can sometimes be waived if you hold a personal Athens login. Athens (www.athensams.net) is an access management system that controls secure access to web based services.[7] Your personal Athens login can usually be obtained through your university, postgraduate library or via this website: www.library.nhs.uk.

> Ask your university or medical school librarian if they can provide you with an Athens login

Evaluating articles

Knowledge of EBM is essential for a good evaluation of the articles you have found. Resources are available to assist your assessment of the quality and usefulness of the articles your literature search has discovered. Websites containing reviews and/or evaluations of past research include the following.

➡ The Bandolier website (www.jr2.ox.ac.uk/bandolier) has a 'knowledge library' which contains abstracts of systematic reviews of treatments, evidence about diagnosis, epidemiology or health economics.

➡ Clinical evidence website (www.clinicalevidence.org) provides details of past research on the efficacy and benefits of treatments as well as highlighting gaps in current research and topics that require further investigation.

➡ Cochrane library (www.thecochranelibrary.com) provides updated reviews of research and references of controlled trials.

Who will help you?

Difficulties often arise when you first perform a literature search. Begin by familiarising yourself with the electronic databases and journal access sites. For practice, search for additional information on one of the topics you are learning about each week. Help will always be available at medical school from other medical students who have already got to grips with the technique or library staff. Ask for help in getting started. Libraries also often hold leaflets that detail the processes involved in literature searches; see if these help.

WRITING YOUR PROJECT

How to structure a report

The same basic structure is used for essays, reports and published articles. The sections described below are in the order in which they should be included. Each section can be subdivided if required.

Abstract

The abstract should be written at the end, but should come right at the beginning of your report. It should contain no new information because it functions as a summary of your entire piece. One or two sentences should be written for each of the following sections. Abstracts are difficult to write; they should usually be no more than 100–300 words long and must be concise.

Introduction

The introduction should explain the topic and its importance, previous or supporting work and what your project was designed to find out.

Methods

Whatever you have done should be explained here. If you performed a literature search, include information on where you searched and what you searched for. If you carried out a piece of research, describe exactly how you did this. This section should allow the reader to exactly replicate what you have done; it is the 'recipe' for your project.

Results

Present the results with no interpretation. Clearly state what you have found. Give the information in a plain but concise way. Do not include opinion or comparison with previous studies.

Discussion

The discussion provides opportunity to comment on results, interpret them and compare them with other studies you have discovered. Provide explanations for these results. Make sure you have answered all questions or completed all tasks that you detailed in your introduction. This section can be subdivided into a discussion of your results, strengths and limitations of your study and suggestions for future work.

Conclusion

The conclusion is a summary of what you wanted to do, what you did and what you have found. Do not include information that is not already introduced.

Appendices

Appendices are used for additional information that is not essential for understanding. For example, you may wish to include some raw data or summaries of published work.

References

Reference the literature you have used or included in your work. References are usually required in the Harvard or Vancouver systems (*see* p. 112). Find out which your university prefers.

Further reading

Further reading sections provide space to include information that the interested reader could obtain but that is not essential for the appreciation of your work.

Planning and preliminary work

Be clear about what you are studying before you start. If you are unsure about the focus of your work you will waste a lot of time gathering irrelevant information. Write down clear objectives, criteria for inclusion and research questions and work from these.

You will often gather huge numbers of papers, containing large quantities of information. Divide your work into topic areas then write these headings down. These can serve as sub-headings in your report. As you read literature, note down the relevant information as referenced bullet points under the appropriate heading. This makes it much easier when you come to write up the final document.

Computer skills

Medical schools provide plenty of access to computers: the university / medical school library, computer rooms and halls of residence (if you are living there). However (controversially), life is much easier if you have your own computer. The internet can be accessed at all the venues listed at computer access points and some universities may also have wireless access around the campus or university buildings.

You are expected to word-process your work. Be competent in using a word processor. Each university will use slightly different software and / or you may have personal favourites. However, most word processors have the same or similar features. Therefore, rather than explaining how to use computer software, this section will explain which computer skills you should master during medical school. Ask the computer technicians at your medical school, university or library if you need assistance. In addition, the computer programs themselves often have superb, searchable help pages that can guide you round the functions of the package. As with most things, the best way to learn how to use computer software is to practise. If you are just starting out, leave plenty of time to familiarise yourself with all the functions of the program when you are compiling your project.

Spelling and grammar

Word processors usually have spelling and grammar checking facilities. You cannot rely solely on these functions to check spelling or grammar, as they do not pick up all errors. For example, the spell checker will not pick up wrong words spelt correctly, for example 'form' instead of 'from'.

The spell checker function uses the computer's inbuilt dictionary. In medicine many words are not present in the generic dictionary. To ensure you spell these words correctly each time, and that the spell checker recognises them as correct, add them to the dictionary as you write. Just make sure you have spelt the word correctly using a medical dictionary before adding it to the computer dictionary.

If there are any words you consistently spell wrong, unless the wrong spelling actually spells another word, you can set the computer to auto-correct words to the correct spelling each time you spell them incorrectly.

Personalising your work

Make the document your own. Use different headings, borders and fonts to highlight titles and important text. However, be careful with use of very elaborate fonts or many different colours; this can make your project look unprofessional and can make the text difficult to read. Generally, use size 10–12 points for main text and either Times New Roman or Arial fonts.

Additional extras

You may need to insert diagrams, tables or figures. Find out how to produce these added extras and how to insert these properly into a written document. If you are inserting photographs, do not use those containing people unless you have explicit written consent from those included in the picture.

Computer programs are available at university to assist you with statistical calculations. Such programs can also help you to produce graphics that represent your results.

Word counts

> All these words just get in the way of what I'm trying to say.[9]

Stick to word counts. Projects and written reports are set for medical students to investigate a topic in depth and demonstrate their writing ability. It is much easier to write a long piece that is full of waffle than a concise document that captures the reader and conveys the same information.

Usually there is a 10% leeway for the word count on either side of the limit. However, check this out with your university. If you exceed this you are unlikely to get the top grade no matter how good your work is. Plan how many words you will use in each section before you start, then stick to this plan.

It is often easier to write too many words and cut them out. If this is how you work, leave plenty of time at the end of your initial writing, as the pruning process is time-consuming.

Make life easier for yourself. Word processing programs usually have a word count function that enables you to make a word count of the whole document or just a highlighted section.

Referencing

The two main referencing systems are Harvard and Vancouver. Your university may prefer one or the other, so find out which one you are required to use.

Be thorough with your referencing. References should allow the reader to easily access the same information you have. Include information on the:

➡ author, editor, organisation (if unknown put *Anon*)
➡ title
➡ edition
➡ place of publication (if a number of locations are listed, write the first in the list)
➡ publisher
➡ volume
➡ page number
➡ year of publication.

Harvard system

The Harvard system cites references by including the author's surname and year of publication in the text. For example, 'Jones (2006) stated that . . .' or '50% of medical students are gorgeous (Cottrell, 2006) . . .'. At the end of the document, in the references section, the list of references used are presented in alphabetical order according to the authors' surnames and chronologically if the same author has published a few pieces.

If an author has published several articles in the same year this is indicated by placing letters, such as a, b, c, against the year. For example, 'Jones (2006a) discovered medical students are wonderful at everything, which was supported by Jones (2006b) finding that they can do nothing wrong'.

For references written by more than one author, only the first author's surname should be included in the text but followed by *et al.* For example, 'Jones *et al.* (2006) . . .'.

You will be able to obtain further information on referencing from your university; however, two templates are given below.

➡ Author Initials (e.g. Jones AP). Year of publication. *Title of the Book*. Edition (e.g. 2nd ed). Location of publication: Publisher.
➡ Author Initials (e.g. Mann D, Hughes K). Year of publication. Title of the article. *Journal name*; **Volume number** (and issue number if required): Page number(s).

Vancouver system

The Vancouver system uses numbers that relate to the references. Numbers are inserted as references are added and must run in order. The reference section then contains a list of references in numerical order. If the same reference is used twice in the same piece, the same number is applied each time. Examples of the Vancouver system can be found throughout this book. For example, 'medical students who choose to read a survival guide[1] are much cleverer than those who do not[2] and they have much more sense.'[3] The references are presented in the format of the following templates.

1 Author Initials (e.g. Cottrell E). *Title of the book*. Edition (e.g. 2nd ed). Location of publication: Publisher; Year of publication.
2 Author Initials (e.g. Bloggs J). Title of the article. *Journal name*. Year of publication; **Volume number** (and issue number if required): Page number(s).
3 Author Initials. Title of web page. Year of publication. (Available at: website address. Accessed (date of download of information).)

Finishing off

Before you finish, ensure your introduction accurately introduces your project. Ensure the conclusion accurately reflects the project and the abstract concisely summarises each section.

Ask someone to proof-read your work. They will often pick up mistakes that you do not notice and can check the work for ease of reading and understanding.

Add the final word count, your name and the title to the front cover of your work. Place the document in a presentation folder or get it bound. A good first impression of your work is helpful.

FURTHER READING

General Medical Council. *Research*. London: General Medical Council; 2002.

Selvanathan SK. The art of the abstract. *StudentBMJ*. 2006; **14**: 70–1.

Tagal J. Difficulties in undergraduate medical research. *The Clinical Teacher*. 2007; **4**: 2–5.

What is evidence based medicine? (Available at: www.jr2.ox.ac.uk/bandolier/painres/download/whatis/ebm.pdf)

CHAPTER 10

Oral presentations

During your medical training you will have to perform oral presentations. Daunting tasks at the best of times, medical school presentations are often assessed. Read on for tips to help get you started and to avoid common pitfalls.

> Take part in departmental teaching or a 'Grand Round', for example, when doing a student-selected component (SSC) project. SSCs require you to focus on a specific disease or patient and to perform some in-depth research around the topic. Therefore the content of your project is detailed and suitable for presentation to doctors. Your SSC tutor may be willing for you to present at these educational meetings and may help you to make the necessary arrangements. Build your confidence in presenting and stand out from other students during assessed presentations. *(Kate Fraser, fourth-year medical student, Manchester)*

You may have to give oral presentations for a number of reasons, to different audiences and on a variety of subjects. However, the basic principles remain the same. Below is a guide to help you.

HOW TO PREPARE

As soon as you know you have to do an oral presentation, find out the topic and start your preparation. Early preparation results in familiarity and will improve your performance.

Write down the information you want to include. Identify pertinent, new or difficult concepts that need explanation and use these to structure your slides/ acetates. To help you to establish the flow and structure of the talk, think about the rules of presentations (and reports):

➡ Say what you are going to say
➡ Say it
➡ Say what you have said

If you are presenting a patient's case, ensure patient-identifiable information is omitted; use initials or fake initials, e.g. 'Mr X'.

Know your topic inside out. Regurgitation of misunderstood information is revealed when you are stumped by a simple question. While writing your presentation, think of at least one question that could arise from each concept. If you cannot answer, do further research.

Do you need visual aids? Only use visual aids that will enhance your presentation, otherwise they serve as a distraction for you and your audience. Which visual aids do you have access to (e.g. projector, flipchart or laptop/computer)? If a number of options are available, decide which you are most confident in using and which is the most convenient. For example, if it is possible you will have to make last-minute changes to your presentation, computer slideshow software is best as you can edit this right up to the start of the presentation. For an interactive presentation the best choices may be acetates or a flipchart. Acetates allow neater writing and projection makes them easier to read. However, they are expensive and a flipchart may be more economical.

If equipment is not kept at the venue of your presentation, find out from where you obtain it and ensure it is not booked by anyone else. You will be nervous enough before giving your presentation without having to worry about equipment.

Ensure the computer software and any storage devices (e.g. flash drive, floppy disk and CD) you use are compatible with the computer you will be presenting from. Slideshow software ensures consistency through using the 'master' function and setting up a template for all your slides (e.g. background and fonts). Some software allows insertion of animations. Take care not to overuse animations, which will make your presentation look tacky. Use animations to clearly emphasise important points.

Know your time limit.[1] Once you have established how much time you have, plan the following:

➡ one slide/acetate per minute
➡ one concept per slide/acetate.
➡ five bullet points per slide/acetate; information will be clearer if you use bullet points rather than sentences.[1]

Grab the audience's attention early or they will lose interest. Make the title catchy and intriguing. Know your audience so you can focus the first few slides on their interests.[2] Use simple, lay language, without jargon, despite your audience, as this will prevent confusion or misunderstanding.[2] If you are presenting a case which was a clinical mystery or dilemma, maintain interest by keeping the audience guessing the diagnosis/conclusion for as long as possible.

Ensure all text is legible. Use large, plain fonts. For computer slideshows, a font size of at least 36 pt should be used for titles and 28 pt for body text.[3] Avoid bad use of colour. Do not use colour combinations that are not easily distinguishable.

Common culprits of illegible fonts are yellow on white and red on dark blue (or vice versa). Colour combinations that work are light (white or yellow) on dark (blue or black) background (or vice versa).

Finally, practise, practise and more practise. The audience will rapidly recognise an unprepared speaker who stumbles around sentences and is unclear. Memorise the presentation; certainly do not let the end of the slideshow come as a surprise to you. Use notes as prompts rather than a script. Do not read directly from your visual aids;[3] they are there for the audience, not you.

PREPARATION ON THE DAY

Electronically back-up your work and have it in two different formats. Collect equipment (when appropriate) early in order to set it up and identify/solve problems.

Wear something comfortable and plain. Do not let your outfit detract from what you are saying. Avoid slogans, they are not professional and will distract the audience. If you are worried about perspiring, wear something that camouflages the telltale signs when you 'talk with your arms'.

DURING THE PRESENTATION

Start your presentation confidently and clearly. This, along with your catchy visual aids (if used) and title, will capture and gain respect from your audience. Speaking loudly and clearly does not amount to shouting. Perfect this balance by performing your presentation to a friend or relative in another room. Hold shaky hands loosely together or lay them on a table.

Emphasise important points using your voice (volume, tone and/or articulation).[3] You may notice verbal tics that you have ('er', 'erm', 'um') and will start to analyse everything you say. Ignore these and carry on regardless.

If you are worried about being distracted by questions mid-way through your talk, state clearly at the beginning that you will ask for questions at the end. If you are confident that questions will not put you off, state that you welcome questions throughout the presentation but ask the audience to put their hand up first.

Think about your positioning. Do not pace around as this can distract and annoy your audience. Do not stand in front of your visual aids. Do not face towards your visual aids as you will be talking to a wall or flipchart and no one will hear you. Computer slideshows can prevent this as you stand away from the projected image but can face the computer screen for prompts.

If you will be explaining diagrams, use a pointer. Waving your hand around or vaguely pointing a finger is unhelpful and looks messy.

Summarise what you have said at the end. Emphasise any take-home messages (no more than three or they will be forgotten) and invite questions at the end.

Finally, remember:

➥ few people enjoy doing presentations
➥ most people are nervous
➥ you rarely look or sound as nervous as you are
➥ prepare and you will be fine.

FURTHER READING

Lowe L. *PowerPoint 2003 for Dummies*. Foster City, CA: IDG Press; 2003.

CHAPTER 11

Let's talk money

Medical students often leave university with varying debts. So how can you obtain money? How to make your money go further? This chapter will guide you to sources of money and give you ideas on how to manage it.

WHY IS MONEY SUCH AN ISSUE FOR MEDICAL STUDENTS?

> Plan well, spend well ... (Pauline Law, first-year graduate medical student, Dundee)

Students are renowned for being poor and many revel in this status. So why is money such an issue for medical students? UK undergraduate medical courses are longer than most other university courses, lasting from four to six years. In addition to the longer course length in years, term times are often extended, especially during clinical years. Medical degrees are demanding of university and personal time. Therefore medical students face a long student life and have little spare time to obtain additional income.[1]

One in six medical students is 'very worried' about debt and nearly two-thirds have an overdraft. Another two-thirds of medical students have at least one credit card owing, on average, over £1000.[2] The average medical graduate owes over £20 000 on leaving university.[3] Further, one in ten owes over £25 000 and some owe over £30 000.[4] These sums roughly equal the entire salary earned as a junior doctor in one year and this debt is rising at a rate exceeding that of inflation.

While medical schools (and all other university faculties) are required to partake in widening participation schemes, the above financial constraints act to work against them. Mature students, graduate students and those from low socio-economic backgrounds are increasingly likely to be deterred from studying medicine because of financial concerns.

Medical students sometimes have difficulty seeking help for money troubles. Despite the presence of university or student union advice centres at each university, medical students cannot always access them; causes include:

➡ Being based at hospitals rather than on campus[5]
➡ Limited opening hours of advice centres coinciding with clinical placements[5]
➡ Generic student advice centres viewed as not appreciating medical student-specific concerns[5]

WHAT WILL YOU SPEND MONEY ON?

Tuition fees

Students who started in 2005/2006 (or before) pay a maximum tuition fee of £1175 per year. This amount should not increase other than with inflation.

The total amount to be paid for tuition fees may seem a lot; however, it represents only about 20% of the cost of your studies. In addition, the tuition fees are 'means-tested', that is, depending on your household or personal income, you may not have to pay the full amount. Consult 'aim higher' (www.aimhigher.ac.uk) for more information.[6]

Students joining medical school from 2006/7 will have to pay tuition fees of up to £3000 a year. Countries within the UK have slightly different tuition fee arrangements and differences occur depending on where you live and where you want to study.

Students in Scotland can expect to pay no more than £2700 plus inflation per year until 2010. Those entering medical school in 2006/7 in Northern Ireland and Wales also have lower maximum values for tuition fees. However, fees move back in line with those for England for the 2007/8 cohort of students. Tuition fees have been frozen up to these maximum amounts until at least 2010, and any rise will only be in line with inflation.

Tuition fees are paid upfront; however, you can get help with this. You can take out a *student loan for fees* to cover the tuition fees. This student loan is borrowed and paid back in the same way as the *student loan for maintenance* (*see* p. 123).[6]

From your fifth year of study, you will not have to pay tuition fees. The final year(s) tuition fees are paid through the NHS bursary scheme or equivalent (*see* p. 126).

Living costs

General and nationally accurate advice on living costs is impossible. Living costs vary with location and type of accommodation; however, you should budget for them. So what may your living costs include?

Accommodation

Individual institutions can provide you with information about accommodation costs in the local area, e.g. average rental, travel and bills. Do not forget to budget all your bills: water, gas, electricity, TV, internet and phone bills. If you live in accommodation that is solely occupied by students, you are exempt from council tax. Total exemption does not occur if you live with non-students; however, you may qualify for a discount. Contact your local council for further information and obtain a certificate from your university to pass on to the council as proof of your student status. If you are in halls, you often have to pay to wash and dry clothes but other bills are included. As soon as you know what accommodation you have, investigate these costs.

Contents insurance

University halls accommodation costs often cover contents insurance; however, if you have particularly valuable possessions or live in private accommodation you will need to protect your belongings with contents insurance. Shop around for the best deal: insurance designed for students can be found (*see* www.endsleigh.co.uk).

Food

Realistically estimate how much your food bill is likely to amount to; perhaps visit a supermarket and add up what you are likely to need if you do not normally do the food shopping. Regard alcohol and meat as treats to reduce cost. Chapter 12 contains more money-saving ideas when buying food.

Socialising

You will want to get to know your new peers. This invariably involves going out and spending money. Budget for socialising expenses as these are likely to occur frequently, especially in the first few weeks.

Clothes

Pre-clinical students can often wear whatever they want. However, in your clinical years you will have to ditch the scruffy clothes and find something presentable, smart and appropriate. 'Work clothes' must be viewed as a necessity; you really cannot turn up to the wards in jeans, trainers and a heavy metal t-shirt.

Travel

Research the cost of public transport. If you own a car, add up the relevant expenditures (*see* Chapter 12).

Payment of pre-existing debts or loans

If you have accumulated debts or loans prior to your medical degree make sure you understand the payment schedules and include them in your budget.

Study-related expenses

These are maximal at the beginning of each term or year. Medical books rarely cost under £20 and are commonly £30–£50. Membership of societies and organisations, and subscriptions to journals, often incur expense. Clinical years bring with them the required 'kit': a white coat and a stethoscope. Studying involves 'disposable' costs such as paper, printing and photocopying. Consider these and budget according to whether you will be using public or personal facilities.

> Skeletons? The anatomy labs are usually full of these, and you can usually have access to them at some point. Don't buy one to take home. They upset cleaning staff if you live in university accommodation! And bus drivers are not too keen on them, either! (*Pauline Law, first-year graduate medical student, Dundee*)
>
> Don't rush out and buy daft bits of kit. You will need a quality stethoscope . . . excellent Christmas present from proud parents and family. (If you shop around you will pay between £40 and £60 for a standard doctor's stethoscope.) (*Pauline Law, first-year graduate medical student, Dundee*)

IMPORTANT INFORMATION

A huge number of websites have been created to assist students to understand and handle their money. Be familiar with the following resources for financial information:

➡ all students (www.studentfinancedirect.co.uk)
➡ students in England (www.dfes.gov.uk/studentsupport)
➡ students in Wales (www.learning.wales.gov.uk/students/ and www.studentfinancewales.co.uk)
➡ students in Scotland (www.saas.gov.uk and www.scotland.gov.uk)
➡ students in Northern Ireland (www.delni.gov.uk and www.education-support.org.uk/students).

STUDENT LOANS

There are two types of student loan you may apply for:

➡ *student loan for fees* – paid straight to your university on your behalf
➡ *student loan for maintenance* – paid into your bank account and intended for living costs.

Student loans are low interest and paid back as you earn. The loans, provided by the government, are relatively non-profit making. The interest paid is linked to inflation. Therefore, in real terms, you pay back roughly what you borrowed.[7] You are expected to pay back the loan once you earn over £15 000 per year.[6] Student loans are paid back at a rate of 9% of your gross, taxable income over the £15,000 threshold. The more you earn, the more you pay back; repayments are not linked to the amount owed. If you lose your job (and income), repayments cease until you reach the threshold again. The income threshold may change in future years so research the correct value at the time you apply for your loan.

Student loan repayments are controlled for you. The Inland Revenue will deduct the money from your salary in the same way in which your national insurance and tax is removed.

Students entering medical school in (or after) 2006 have the benefit that any student loan outstanding, 25 years after the April your course finishes, will be written off. Exceptions do apply, investigate this before you take out the loan.[6]

The amount of loan you are entitled to depends upon factors such as:[6]

➥ living at home or not
➥ living in London or not
➥ your household income or, if you are an independent student, your personal income (it is 'means-tested')
➥ receiving maintenance grant or not: students receiving a maintenance grant receive less student loan; however, the grant makes up this deficit. Such students are advantaged as there is less loan to pay back.[6]

Although student loans are 'means-tested', all eligible students are given 75% of the maximum loan. Only the remaining 25% is means-tested. However, if you are eligible for the maximum loan, you do not have to borrow the sum in its entirety.

There is no upper age limit for student loan for fees.[6] This assists mature and graduate students to enter university, in concordance with widening participation schemes.

MAINTENANCE GRANTS

Maintenance grants were introduced in 2006. They provide monies for full-time students from lower income families. Eligibility for the maintenance grant thus depends upon either your household income or, if you are an independent student, your personal income (including your partner's income if applicable). Depending on the level of this income you may receive part or all of £2700 per year, plus any rise with inflation. A third of the maintenance grant is paid at the start of each term.[6]

Students receiving the full £2700 maintenance grant and who are on courses charging tuition fees in excess of this must get extra help from their university. Many universities have taken this one step further and have also pledged to bridge the deficit for those who are not entitled to the full £2700 maintenance grant.[7] Make sure you find out your institution's position on this.

APPLYING FOR STUDENT LOANS AND MAINTENANCE GRANTS

Applications for both student loans and the maintenance grant are covered by one form. Application forms are usually available from March and a firm offer of a place is not required to apply. Apply for your money online at www.studentfinancedirect.co.uk. This website also contains information on available support for students entering higher education in the coming year, instructions for application and a tool to estimate the amount of money you are likely to be entitled to. Apply as early as you can so you know what money you are entitled to in plenty of time to budget.[7]

When making your application you have to provide your local authority with your National Insurance number and birth certificate/passport. The local authority will inform you of any other documents they require to process your application.

Other useful websites include:
➡ Student Loans Company (www.slc.co.uk)
➡ for students living in England (www.studentfinancedirect.co.uk)
➡ for students living in Wales (www.studentfinancewales.co.uk)
➡ for students living in Scotland (www.saas.gov.uk)
➡ for students living in Northern Ireland (www.delni.gov.uk).

STUDENT BANK ACCOUNTS

You need a bank account. High street banks provide great student packages, some offer joining incentives such as free student rail cards, CDs or money. However, investigate the overdraft facilities, interest rates and graduate accounts when choosing your student bank account.

Overdraft limits and interest rates vary from bank to bank. They sometimes vary within a bank as you progress through university. Often, your overdraft limit will increase with your student years. However, it is important you understand that if your first year overdraft is £1000 and it increases in your second year to £1500, this does not mean you can withdraw £2500 below zero. You can only access a further £500 in the second year. Overdraft agreements upon graduation also vary. Although you should consider graduate arrangements when choosing a student bank account, you are able to change banks whenever you like. So watch out for offers and packages and change banks if a better deal can be obtained elsewhere.

Graduate bank accounts can be beneficial. Some offer mortgages, loans and interest-free overdrafts for a fixed period of time following your graduation. These can help to get you on your feet when you start work.

Other factors to consider when choosing a bank are:
➡ Where is the nearest branch?
➡ Is it near to your campus, medical school or accommodation? Bank employees may be more sympathetic to (or tolerant of) students if the branch is on a university campus.
➡ Do you want a bank with internet access and/or postal facilities?

In order to obtain a student bank account you may need to be a permanent UK resident (have been in UK for at least three years before your course starts), be studying on an Honours-degree course of three or more years in length or have an unconditional offer letter or a UCAS acceptance letter for a full-time Honours degree course.

> Does your chosen university have scholarships or bursaries on offer? When is the closing date? Do they require you to apply before they offer you a place? Don't be afraid to apply. Be positive but be realistic. To gain a scholarship you will need to demonstrate not only need but what unique characteristics you are bringing to the university, faculty or campus. (*Pauline Law, first-year graduate medical student, Dundee*)

SCHOLARSHIPS, GRANTS AND BURSARIES

Universities offer scholarships based on various criteria. They may be offered to students who:

➥ are from certain social environments
➥ achieve high marks in their pre-university exams
➥ perform well at interview
➥ demonstrate sporting excellence or music talent.
➥ perform well in a university exam.

Contact your university for details of the scholarships it offers.

If your medical school charges more than £2700 for annual tuition fees, it is required to provide financial support to those receiving the full maintenance grant of £2700, in order to bridge the shortfall; that is, universities must provide up to £300. This money may be awarded as a bursary, scholarship or by some other means; contact your institution for specific information. Some medical schools offer bursaries amounting to more than the minimum sum required. For example, medical students entering Oxford University or Imperial College in 2006 from low-income families were offered bursaries resulting in an income of up to £4000 a year. Other universities offer course-cost bursaries, non-course-related bursaries and sports passes.

> Scholarships or bursaries can be found on the internet. Not everyone will be eligible for each, as some are very specific in whom they will give money to. Don't waste their time – and your stamps – if you don't fit the criteria specified. (*Pauline Law, first-year graduate medical student, Dundee*)

Universities have been urged to clearly advertise the bursaries on offer. Therefore you should be able to easily access such information prior to and while you are at medical school.

Useful sources of grant, bursary, scholarship and award information include:
- ➡ Hotcourses (www.hotcourses.com)
- ➡ Uniburse: the bursary information and student portal (www.uniburse.com)
- ➡ Royal Medical Benevolent Fund (www.rmbf.org)
- ➡ Royal Medical Foundation (www.royalmedicalfoundation.org)
- ➡ BMA charities: gives assistance to doctors and their dependants at times of crisis and makes some one-off grants and occasionally interest-free loans (email info.bmacharities@bma.org.uk)
- ➡ Educational Grants Advisory Service (www.egas-online.org/fwa/).

NHS BURSARY

English domiciled medical students, who started on or after 1 September 1998 qualify for NHS financial support in their fifth and further years of study. This support is means-tested. You or your parents, spouse or partner (as applicable) are required to provide information on your household income. You may be eligible for an NHS bursary and help with tuition fees. Students on four-year graduate entry courses are eligible for NHS bursaries, tuition fee assistance and up to 50% of the full loan from the second year.

The bursary is intended for day to day living costs. The amount you are awarded is the amount you will receive, as Income Tax and National Insurance are not deducted.

Once you reach the appropriate year of your course to receive the NHS bursary, your medical school will inform the NHS Pensions Agency Students Grants Unit (SGU). The SGU will send you a 'Bursary pack' that you have to complete and return with supporting documentation (when applicable).

You may be eligible for extra payments in addition to your bursary; reasons for this include:
- ➡ extra weeks' attendance
- ➡ older students (over 26 years before first academic year)
- ➡ dependants' allowances, childcare allowance, disabled student allowance and care-givers allowance.

Some students entering their fifth year of study in 2005/6 encountered huge delays in obtaining money from the NHS SGU (www.nhsstudentgrants.co.uk). As a result the system was changed. However, you are advised to assist rapid and efficient processing of your application and documents by returning your form(s) promptly. Ensure you have access to other money until your allocation arrives in your bank account.

A similar bursary is available to Scottish medical students, the Scottish Executive Health Department bursary (*see* www.saas.gov.uk/home.htm).

TRAVEL ALLOWANCE COSTS

Normal daily travel between home and medical school is not eligible for reimbursement. However, additional travel expenses may be claimed. If your placements are further than (or incur costs in excess of) your normal travel from home to university, you may qualify for reimbursement from the NHS SGU (www.nhsstudentgrants.co.uk). Reimbursement covers the cost of the cheapest mode of transport (usually public transport). If public transport is not an option (unavailable/unsuitable), claims for the use of your own vehicle can only be accepted following prior agreement from your medical school.

BANK LOANS

High-street banks may offer loans to medical students, for example:
- professional trainee loans – repayments occur after graduation
- graduate loans (for graduate medical students).

Money can be borrowed as a lump sum or in instalments. Conditions apply for bank loans; for example, some banks do not provide loans to first-year students. Investigate up-to-date loan information, terms and conditions before using this resource.

CAREER DEVELOPMENT LOANS

Career development loans (CDL) are managed by the Department for Education and Skills (DfES); however, they are expensive. You may be eligible for a CDL if you are ordinarily a resident in England, Scotland or Wales and intend to work within the EU, Iceland, Norway or Liechtenstein once you graduate. Consider a CDL if you are unable to get support from your local authority and have no other access to funds. The CDL should cover your course fees and living expenses; maximal sums of money are awarded to individuals who have been out of work for at least three months. To apply you are required to complete an application form for the bank of your choice. For further information go to your local job centre or talk to your career adviser. You can also obtain a CDL application pack by phoning 0800 585505. Also, see the website www.lifelonglearning.dfes.gov.uk/cdl.

PARENTS

Unfortunately, those students deemed to be 'dependent' on their parents (read parents, guardians and/or carers) and whose parents' income is above the threshold for means-tested money will receive less student loan and will have to pay maximum tuition fee costs. Unless you have your own funds, or enough time to work, you are likely to need financial assistance. If your parents have the money, they may help you out; however, if they do not have funds you will need to pursue the other options in this chapter. How you arrange financial help from your parents is entirely personal so no more will be said. This source of help is included for completion.

HARDSHIP LOAN AND ACCESS TO LEARNING FUNDS

Hardship loans may be an option if you have already accepted the maximum student loan you are entitled to and have received the first instalment. Up to £500 per year in five divided sums may be awarded. To qualify for a hardship loan you must prove financial hardship. The loan is repaid in the same way as the student loan.

Access to learning funds or financial contingency funds (Wales) are available from universities to provide extra financial support for students with a low income. The application involves a form on which you detail your income and expenditure. Based on this information, your payment will be calculated. Payments may be given in lump sums or instalments. The money may be a loan or a non-repayable grant. Priority is often given to mature students, students with children (especially lone parents) and final-year students. Contact your university for further information.

JOBS

> Remember that you are at medical school to become a doctor and there is no point struggling to obtain money unless you pass the exams. Don't sacrifice revision for working. It is the drinking time that will have to suffer. You should forward plan your paid work around exam periods by arranging annual leave or unpaid leave for at least the week before your exams. (*Pauline Law, first-year graduate medical student, Dundee*)

Modern life provides little for free. The only source of extra money for many students is part-time work. Part-time jobs include holiday jobs and regular evening or weekend work. Consider flexible jobs; your spare time in which you are available to work may not be predictable or stable. Possible jobs are obviously vast and varied; however, a few serve to provide an income and are helpful for your degree (*see below*).

Go to www.bma.org.uk/ap.nsf/Content/studentsandtaxcodes for information on the tax you should and should not be liable to pay.

Healthcare-related jobs

Healthcare-related jobs include:
➡ healthcare assistant

➡ care worker
➡ domestic.

Healthcare assistants and care workers usually work in hospitals and care homes, respectively. Duties include washing, dressing and feeding patients and residents. These jobs teach you:

➡ how to interact with older and/or sick people
➡ the routines of a hospital
➡ how to use basic medical equipment (blood pressure machine, thermometer, the beds)
➡ about death
➡ some basic knowledge on medical conditions and procedures; depending upon your experience you may also perform clinical skills such as recording ECGs (electrical tracing of the heart), applying dressings and removing sutures, clips or drains.

Healthcare assistant and care worker posts can often be obtained through an agency or 'nurse bank'. The 'nurse bank' is usually hospital- or trust-based and consists of a number of full-time and part-time nurses (qualified and not) who are willing to work extra shifts when additional staff are required. You can work solely as a bank nurse, without being employed on an individual ward. Agencies are similar, but are profit-making companies external to the trust/hospital. Often you get paid more but may be asked to work anywhere in the local area. Because agencies charge a lot for the hire of their nurses, they are only used if the hospital is desperate, therefore work may not be predictable.

The benefits of working for a nurse bank or agency are:

➡ you decide when and where you want to work to some extent
➡ you can move around wards, hospitals and or homes so you will learn the routines and roles of many clinical environments
➡ acquisition of skills, such as interaction with total strangers
➡ ability to mould your work to apply to your current university module.

The disadvantages of working for a nurse bank or agency are:

➡ work is not guaranteed
➡ you may be asked to work in wards you do not know or like
➡ availability of work may become increasingly unreliable as the NHS cuts costs and uses bank and agency nurses less often.

If nursing work does not appeal but you want experience of a hospital setting before entering your clinical years, think about becoming a domestic assistant. Domestics are known by many different titles, including housekeeping assistants and hotel services. Domestics keep the ward clean and provide refreshments for patients. You will learn the layout of clinical environments and will gain experience in interacting with patients.

Write to your local hospital for information on such vacancies.

Research

Research takes time and medical professionals are busy. Therefore, if you are interested in spending your holiday(s) searching for literature or collating data, consider helping with a research project. The pay is usually poor; however, you will learn research skills, gain a deeper understanding of the topic being researched and perhaps even publish an article as a result (and thus enhance your future job applications). Information on researchers looking for help may be posted on notice boards in and around the medical school and hospital. Alternatively, if a particular topic interests you, ask the relevant consultant if any research is ongoing that you could participate in.

Phlebotomy

Why not practise taking blood while earning money? Join the team of phlebotomists at your local hospital and set yourself up for future success with even the most difficult of veins. Contact your local hospital for more information.

Serving the public

Jobs do not have to be medical-related to be useful. Working as a waiter/waitress, behind a bar or cashier provides exposure to the general public. This will increase your confidence in speaking with strangers and will give you experience in dealing with complaints and unhappy customers, which is useful for medicine. This type of work is often easy to come by. However, working times can be long, antisocial and exhausting, especially if you are working in a bar or club.

Medical school

Medical schools often provide the opportunity for you to earn some 'pocket money' if you are willing to assist with practical exams of other years, take prospective and new students on tours of the hospital/medical school and attend recruitment fairs. Other than financial gain, you will benefit from the experience of exams from 'the other side'. Taking students on tours and attending fairs allows you to practise your communication skills with many new people.

WELSH STUDENTS

An Assembly Learning Grant may be available if you are from a low-income family, are a full-time student studying at a publicly funded college in the UK and are normally a resident in Wales. The grant does not need to be repaid. See the website www.learning.wales.gov.uk/students.

SCOTTISH STUDENTS

In December 1999, the Cubie Report[8] was published in response to tuition fees in Scotland. The Committee of Inquiry recommended that tuition fees for Scottish students should be abolished and continuation of grants for further education students should occur. It also recommended the introduction of Wider Access Bursaries and Mature Student Bursaries for disadvantaged students and additional support for lone parents, mature students with children and students with disabilities. These changes would only apply to Scottish students studying in Scottish universities, not English students studying in Scotland.[9] As a result of The Cubie report, Scottish students who are/will be studying in a Scottish university may have a different financial situation to that described above. You may be eligible for a means tested bursary in addition to a partly means tested student loan. Contact your university finance office for more information.

The Graduate Endowment Scheme for Higher Education applies to Scottish graduates (from Scotland or anywhere in the EU) who, after completing their first degree, have to pay a sum of around £2000 to help future generations of disadvantaged students. The payment made by graduates is offset by the benefits they gain from their degree. The following students are not expected to pay into the scheme:
- mature students
- lone parents
- disabled students.

Eligible students apply to pay the Graduate Endowment while applying to the Students Award Agency for Scotland (SAAS) for maintenance support. Post-graduation you have until the following April to decide whether you will pay the Graduate Endowment upfront or through a student loan repayment system. If you are liable to pay the Graduate Endowment you may be eligible for an additional student loan to cover this payment.

If you are under 25 years old on the first day of the academic year of your course, are from a low-income background and live in Scotland you may be eligible for a non-repayable Young Students' Bursary. Mature students may also be eligible for a similar award, the Mature Students' Bursary. It is the higher education institutions rather than the SAAS that award these bursaries; however, you can visit the SAAS website (www.saas.gov.uk/home.htm) or the institution websites for further information.

A Young Students' Outside Scotland Bursary may be available to you if you are a Scottish student from a low-income family who is studying at a UK institution. This bursary is means-tested.

You may be able to seek help from the Carnegie Trust for university fees if you cannot obtain help elsewhere, are of Scottish birth or extraction and/or have had two years' education at a secondary school in Scotland. You cannot obtain assistance for maintenance costs from this source. The Carnegie Trust also offers a Vacation Scholarship Scheme that provides funds for eligible students to undertake research during their summer vacation. Consult the website www.carnegie-trust.org for more information and application forms.

SPECIAL CIRCUMSTANCES

Students with children

If you have children and are in full-time higher education you may be eligible for financial assistance. A brief summary of the help available will be provided here but consult your Local Authority for further information. *See* the website www.dfes.gov. uk/studentsupport/students/lon_lone_parents.shtml.

Childcare Allowance is available to students with dependant children aged 14 or below (or 16 or below if the child(ren) has(have) special educational needs) on the first day of the academic year. This award is means-tested and will cover a maximum of 85% of the costs of childcare at a registered or approved childcare provider. Monies provided by the childcare grant depend on the cost of the childcare and your income. Application occurs at the same time you apply for your student loan. You will need to state the cost of childcare and provide evidence of payment. Make sure you obtain and retain all receipts.

The Single Parent Addition is an allowance that is available to single students who have a dependant child or children. This cannot be received in addition to the Older Students' Allowance (*see* 'Mature students' section). For more information consult the NHS SGU website www.nhsstudentgrants.co.uk.

Full-time students with dependant children, who are not already receiving the Lone Parents' Grant, may qualify for Parents' Learning Allowance. The allowance is income-assessed. Applications occur through the local authority.

Apply to the Inland Revenue for the Child Tax Credit, which has replaced the Dependants' Grant for children. If you are entitled to full Child Tax Credit, and are not receiving Working Tax Credit, your children can receive free school meals. The amount of Child Tax Credit you may be entitled to is dependent on your income. *See* the website www.inlandrevenue.gov.uk/taxcredits.

If you are living in Wales, are in higher education and have children, you may qualify for the Assembly Learning Grant. The Assembly Learning Grant is intended to help cover the cost of books, equipment, travel and childcare while you are studying. *See* the website www.learning.wales.gov.uk.

Finally, some universities offer financial assistance to students with children. Contact your university finance office or student support centre for further information.

Students with adult dependants

If you live with an adult (e.g. a husband, wife or partner) who is financially dependent on you and you are in full-time higher education, you may qualify for the Adult Dependants' Grant. The grant depends on your total incomes. Apply through your local authority.

Students with disabilities

Disabled students in higher education may be entitled to a Disabled Student Allowance (DSA). The DSA is not means-tested but based on a needs assessment. It is intended to cover extra study costs resulting from your special needs; for example, a support worker and/or mentor, longer deadlines, information technology and help in organising work and routines. Payments are managed by the local authority (England and Wales), the SAAS (Scotland) or the Education and Libraries Board (Northern Ireland).[7] The allowance is non-repayable. Other benefits available to disabled students can be investigated on the Skill websites www.skill.org.uk and www.dfes.gov.uk/studentsupport/formsandguides/index.shtml (information, forms, guidance and links to other sources of help for students with disabilities).

Mature students

If you are 26 years old before 1 September of the year your course starts, you may qualify for the Older Students' Allowance from the NHS SGU. The allowance depends on your age before the start of your course, but does not increase annually throughout the course. You cannot receive this allowance in addition to the Single Parent Addition, even if you qualify for both. *See* the website www.nhsstudentgrants.co.uk.

Graduate students

Financial support for postgraduate students is not compulsory. Consult your university to discuss any funding it provides. You may be eligible for some of the awards discussed in this chapter. Thoroughly investigate sources of funding such as access to learning funds, scholarships, grants and bursaries.

> Funding is really difficult for graduates and no one seems to want to help. (*Pauline Law, first-year graduate medical student, Dundee*)

Graduate students on traditional undergraduate degree courses may be eligible for a British Medical Association (BMA) grant, a BMA Medical Education Trust Grant. Only a limited number of awards are available for students and applications must be made a year in advance of the award being given. Applications will be assessed on the basis of academic merit and financial need. For details on this grant and information on eligibility and how to apply email info.bmacharities@bma.org.uk.

SAVING MONEY WHILE YOU STUDY

Budgeting

The horrifying word 'budget' will be mentioned repeatedly in this chapter. However, budgeting helps you to manage your money and can help you to save it, too.

Budgeting may be as popular among students as eating soup off a dissection table. It does not conform to the crazy image that most students strive to achieve. However, being left with £5 to spend for the last seven weeks of term is not all that crazy in reality. Money will never be in endless supply. Learning how to budget now will prepare you for looking after your money later in life. So where do you start?

First, work out all your income.

➡ *Lump sums at the beginning of each term (e.g. student loan, maintenance grants)*: Remember these lump sums are calculated by dividing your annual entitlement equally among the three terms. However, your terms are usually not equal in length. You may wish to budget the actual money you will receive at the beginning of each term or 'borrow' some from future terms to get you through the longest first term (bear in mind that 'borrowing' is from your own account so you may have to use overdraft for this).

➡ *Jobs*: If you have not got regular work organised, do not rely on this income. There is no guarantee you will find a job and/or have time to work. If you do not have a regular income, view additional money as a bonus with which you can treat yourself.

➡ *Overdraft*: You may wish to budget the available money in your overdraft. However, doing this will leave you without any 'emergency money'.

➡ *Other income*: Do you have a scholarship, money from family or income from a partner?

Next, work out your likely outgoings.

➡ Consider what you will spend money on: research the relevant costs and note each down.

➡ Do you have a hobby/interest that involves subscription charges or consumables?

➡ Do you want to put money aside for holidays or presents (e.g. birthday or festivals)?

You can get assistance with the above steps from a budget calculator (*see* www. aimhigher.ac.uk/student_finance/cost_of_living_calculator.cfm). Once you have worked out your income and likely expenditure, subtract the expenditure from the income. If this results in a positive number, congratulations! If not, you are on the path to debt before you have even started. Look at your income and expenditure again and find ways of increasing your income (difficult) or cutting back on the expenditure.

Once your budget is in positive balance, submit it to paper. Obviously, personal preference should be followed, but one way that works will be described for beginners.

➡ Construct a spreadsheet or written table containing the columns that represent the major classes of expenditure (*see* Figure 11.1):

 – Set expenditure (may be allocated as a lump sum or regular instalments): bills; food; transport; rent.
 – Flexible expenditure (non-reliable expenditure should be paid in as lump sums to allow for large payments at the beginning of term): socialising money; course-related expenditure; clothes.
 – Have an 'extra' column for unexpected or unspent money. Use this as guilt-free money for treats or to cover costs you had not budgeted for (remember to add these into your budget for the next term if they are recurring).

➡ Calculate the proportion of your income you will attribute to each column.
➡ Calculate a fortnightly minimum target your money can drop down to. This allows for an expensive week followed by a cheap week without blowing the budget.
➡ As you spend money, remove the value from the appropriate column. If you are using a credit card you can remove the sum of money from the appropriate column and place it into a 'credit card' column. You can then pay the credit card bill out of the 'credit card' column.

 – Every time money is removed from your bank record how much and details of the expenditure.
 – Save money without realising it by rounding up expenditures to the nearest pound. Each time you spend money you will be subtracting a few pence that has not been spent. At the end of the term, check your budget for what money you think you have, against the money in the bank and the difference is what you have saved. After a term this can be enough for a holiday (honestly).

Date	Description	Spending	Target	Bills	Food	Transport	Rent	Extra	Credit card
01/09/2006	Student loan and money from parents	£900.00	£760.00	£150.00	£280.00	£150.00	£2,000.00	£0.00	£0.00

Figure 11.1 Sample of a written budget (values are examples, calculate your own).

Budgeting is a dynamic process. Change it accordingly as you learn the costs of daily living. The main concepts are to be aware of:

➡ what money you have
➡ how long the money you have has to last for
➡ what you have to spend your money on

Books

Medical degree textbooks are expensive; save money by:

➡ going to or organising your own book fairs and/or second-hand bookshops

➡ using library books

➡ taking advantage of offers from medical organisations; they often provide free books or offer reduced prices for their members.

> I wish I knew in the first year that you don't need to buy every textbook that they tell you to. Some people learn so much better by different textbooks, and I think some lecturers assume we have lots of money.
> *(Rachel Boyce, first-year medical student, Aberdeen)*

Journals

It is unfeasible to subscribe to each journal you like and use. University libraries provide access to a good selection of electronic journals (which can be accessed over the internet) and/or paper journals. Save money by:

➡ reading electronic journals on the computer screen, rather than printing them

➡ only printing/copying relevant pages

➡ setting photocopiers to reduce two pages to fit onto one A4 sheet.

Transport

The cost of public transport varies hugely. Week, month or year travel cards can greatly reduce expense. Using your own transport is often not the cheapest mode of transport (*see* Chapter 12). If you use your car, share lifts. Take turns to drive or regularly give someone a lift and share the petrol money.

The cheapest and healthiest mode of transport is walking. Walk to university if it is possible and safe. It may take additional time but this often clears your mind of the day's worries and/or clarifies confusions arising from the day's learning. The exercise will also burn off last night's beer and kebab!

Biking into university is an option. However, ensure there is somewhere secure to leave your bicycle. In areas where biking is common, so is bicycle theft. Do not use a top-of-the-range mountain bike, purchase the cheapest bicycle you can to reduce losses in the event of a theft.

Accommodation

The cheapest accommodation is living at home. This option may not be possible or, in your eyes, reasonable. However, if your parents live close it is a great way of saving money. Your parents may also be pleased because they will know you are safe.

If you live away from home, research all the accommodation options available. With increasing cost, there is usually increasing quality or convenience. Decide how much you are willing to save based on what you will miss out on in cheaper accommodation.

If you are sharing accommodation, reach an arrangement among your house-mates with regards to buying washing up liquid, toilet roll, coffee, sugar, etc. There is no point having eight bottles of washing up liquid in your kitchen.

Food

> Shop carefully. Have a budget. Ensure food is nutritious and balanced. You are a medical student, you have a duty to your body to keep it a mean, lean learning machine. *(Pauline Law, first-year graduate medical student, Dundee)*

How to save money on food

➡ Do not eat takeaway every night. It is not healthy or cheap.

➡ Do not only buy branded products. Value ranges contain many products such as tinned tomatoes, fresh fruit and vegetables, pasta, rice, beans and bread. They may not be identical to popular brands; however, there is often nothing wrong with the quality.

➡ Take a packed lunch and drinks. Buying a cooked lunch or sandwich plus a drink every lunch time can easily add up to over £10 every week, even at student establishments.

➡ Take advantage of offers. Supermarkets always have offers on different food, drink and household items. Work out how much you will save and if it is a good deal, and you normally buy the item, make the purchase.

➡ Familiarise yourself with each supermarket in your local area and frequent the cheapest.

➡ Buy food online. There is often a delivery charge for home shopping, but if you split this money between your flatmates it may not amount to anymore than a bus fare or petrol. Impulse buys are also avoided.

➡ Cook large quantities and create your own ready meals at a fraction of the price by putting the excess in the fridge/freezer.

➡ Only shop once a week. Do not be tempted to go back for forgotten items, you inevitably see and buy something else you fancy.

SOURCES OF FURTHER HELP, ADVICE AND SERVICES

Professional Medical Finance

As a doctor, your earnings will be several million over your career. For this reason, you need to ensure that all your financial products are appropriate for your situation. Professional Medical Finance (PMF) (www.freefees.co.uk) is a company run by doctors that aims to give back to other doctors as much as they possibly can. PMF claim you will not find better rewards elsewhere. PMF praises itself in knowing which products (e.g. bank accounts, personal loans, mortgages and protection products) doctors need at the different stages of their career, and helping to provide them.

money4medstudents

A website called money4medstudents (www.money4students.org) has been created by a partnership between the British Medical Association (BMA), Council of Heads of Medical Schools (CHMS), the National Association of Student Money Advisers (NASMA) and the Royal Medical Benevolent Fund (RMBF). The website contains links that will provide help and information if you are trying to find ways to increase your income, get a loan or curb your spending. Easy to follow features, such as a budget planner and debt calculator, will be useful resources that will help you to follow advice outlined in this chapter. Also available on money4medstudents is an online money advice clinic from which you can obtain individualised advice for your own financial situation.

Royal Bank of Scotland Student Living Index 2004

Information on costs of living in different universities across the UK and experiences of individual students can be found in the *Royal Bank of Scotland Student Living Index*. This document also contains tips for saving money. Download this useful resource from the website http://image.guardian.co.uk/sysfiles/Education/documents/2004/08/23/bank.pdf.

Wesleyan Medical Sickness

Have you ever thought about what you would do if accident or illness prevented you from working and earning an income? The Medical Career Protector from the Wesleyan Assurance Society is specifically designed for medical students and doctors. Exclusively provided through Wesleyan Medical Sickness, it is designed to protect your income should you suffer loss of earnings as a result of illness or accident. As a final-year medical student Wesleyan Medical Sickness can arrange cover for you free of charge, as they understand it is cover that you may not be able to afford. Then when you qualify as a doctor, a monthly fee will help to provide the cover you will need in the early years of your career. Wesleyan Medical Sickness has a dedicated team of Student Liaison Managers covering medical schools across the UK who can provide information about and access to the cover.

Wesleyan Medical Sickness has been addressing the needs of medics since 1884 and is part of the Wesleyan Assurance Society, one of the oldest and financially strong mutual organisations in the UK. It also offers a wide range of insurance products for students, covering elective travel, motor and personal possessions; *see* the website www.wesleyanmedicalsickness.co.uk.

A FEW FINAL WORDS

All the above information is intended as a guide to what is available; it should not be used as a recommendation or as personal or definitive advice and the author cannot be held responsible for any financial difficulties you may encounter in the future.

You are responsible for the financial decisions and movements you make. If you are unclear about your financial situation or require financial support, seek help from your university promptly.

Never provide false information when completing forms for financial support or loans – it is an offence. Keeping your financial providers up-to-date with your circumstances is your responsibility.

Do not get bogged down by worrying about money. Providing you are sensible with your cash and you pass your exams, you will soon be earning a more-than-adequate wage to pay back student loans and overdrafts. Enjoy yourself within your financial limits.

FURTHER READING

www.aimhigher.ac.uk/student_financc/2006_onwards.cfm
www.egas-online.org
Medical student finance section of the British Medical Association website www.bma.org.uk
www.nusonline.co.uk/info/money
www.studentmoney.org
www.studentpages.com
www.studentuk.com

CHAPTER 12

Life away from medicine

Establishing a healthy work–life balance is difficult but crucial. What are the considerations for life away from medicine? What are the different types of accommodation available to you? What can you do with your 'spare time'? How can you stay happy and healthy? What facilities are available for students with families and children? Read on for tips to prevent medicine taking over your life.

ACCOMMODATION

You may reside in various types of accommodation while at university. In the first year, many students choose to live in university halls of residence ('halls'). Below are the main choices for accommodation you have to choose from.

➡ *Living at home*: a possibility if you already live within one hour of the university buildings.
➡ *University halls of residence, university flat or university house*: more expensive but better regulated than private accommodation.
➡ *Privately rented flat or house*: the Student Accommodation Office may provide you with a list of approved landlords or schemes to get you started.
➡ *Owned house or flat*: an option for a minority of medical students.
➡ *Couple and family accommodation*: university couple and family accommodation is not readily available; however, the Student Accommodation Office may help couples and families find appropriate accommodation in the area.

> For many years my passions oscillated between two poles: studying medicine and the music scene at university, along with its concomitant social life. Located at a distance of merely 500 yards from one another, both crystallised the occupations of my first year at university. In a typical week I moved between a circle of friends in the music rooms, clubs and bars of the Student Union to the fascinating, yet completely engrossing, world of the Old Medical School building. My recreational pursuits were communal; my intellectual pursuits individual. The gulf was pronounced:

friends rarely joined me as I extracted layers of adipose tissue from my cadaver in the dissecting room, and the books I obtained from the medical library never accompanied me to the Union.

During my pre-clinical years it was hectic, yet not impossible to juggle my two mistresses, but this is becoming increasingly difficult. On several occasions I have been caught being unfaithful to one or the other. As a student coming to university you have the opportunity to experience many new things. Some may stay out all night, live with flatmates or try alcohol. Despite this, for many, the prerogative remains to obtain a degree. In my opinion one of the biggest challenges facing medical students today is living the 'normal' university life of peers from other courses whilst being put through the paces of a medical degree.

Undoubtedly, medical students have to grow up much faster than their colleagues: unable to skip their first lecture or go in an hour late after a heavy night because they are expected to attend an 8 am X-ray meeting. Naturally, many medical students find it challenging to cope with the pressures that co-exist with studying medicine whilst getting to know peers from other faculties. This may explain why medics often choose to share accommodation. Indeed, a published study showed that medical students who lived off-campus were more likely to drop out during their first year.[1] This finding highlights the influence of wider social integration on academic progression.

Without doubt it is often helpful to have fellow medics at hand to recall the tenth cranial nerve, but after spending the whole day in a hospital teaching environment, is it not healthy to spend some time away from our mistress? Medics should strive to find the narrow balance of work and play. *(Vishnu Madhok, fourth-year medical student, Dundee)*

When choosing a medical school, consider the accommodation on offer as this may be a deciding factor in your application. Wherever you go two resources may be helpful.

➥ *Student accommodation office/services*: source of help, support and contacts for anything accommodation related; if they cannot help they usually know someone who can.

➥ *Disabilities office/officer/adviser/coordinator*: if you have any form of disability that may affect the accommodation you require (e.g. guide dog, wheelchair), seek assistance and support from here.

Halls

If you live in halls for the first year, which I recommend, you will get to know people on other courses. This widens your perspective away from just medicine. *(Zoe Cowan, first-year medical student, Leicester)*

Providing you fulfil the terms and conditions of your university (e.g. application deadlines, no previous university accommodation) you are usually guaranteed a place in university accommodation during your first year, and this is usually a university hall of residence. Look up the terms and conditions well in advance. As you progress through your course university accommodation is less available but still worth a try if it is your preference.

Information on halls of residence will be provided when you accept an offer of a university placement, usually around April of the year you will be studying. Information can be accessed in advance from the university or its website.

Look around various accommodation before you select your choice. Universities often hold accommodation open days. If you cannot attend these arrange a viewing independently with the university.

Deadlines for applications for accommodation vary between universities, but most lie around May/June. Check this out when you receive the accommodation information. Apply for your favourite residences but appreciate you cannot be guaranteed your first choice; so think carefully about all the choices you make. You may have to pay a deposit with your application.

Along with your choice of accommodation, you may be required to provide personal information such as your age, hobbies, ideal flatmates, bedtime and smoking habits. The information you provide is used to match you to like-minded people (if possible).

Accommodation is usually allocated from May onwards. However, students often have very different circumstances (e.g. waiting for exam results, have taken a gap year, postgraduate), so this time varies. Many universities wait until A-level and Scottish Higher results are published before allocating accommodation. Students applying to university through the UCAS 'clearing' system may not be successful in getting university accommodation; however, allocation is attempted. If no accommodation is available the university should provide you with information on temporary alternatives until a solution is found.

In most cases you will be able to move into your halls the Saturday before the term begins. This enables you to settle in, get to know your flatmates and find your way around before the hard slog (and hard partying) starts. Halls often arrange socials during the first few nights to break the ice between new residents.

Types of hall available

Even if you have decided that hall living is for you, the decisions do not end there. A number of different halls should be considered based on the facilities they offer.

➡ *On-campus or off-campus*: on-campus halls may not be as convenient as they sound for medical students spending the majority of their time at clinical placements away from the university campus. If you choose off-campus halls, ensure your routes to the university or placements are safe and relatively short.

➡ *Single, twin or triple rooms*: you may have strong views about sharing a room with other people. Make sure you know about the presence of twin/triple rooms prior to submitting your application.

➡ *Catered, part-catered or self-catered*: this decision boils down to your confidence in the kitchen. Part-catered halls either provide breakfast or breakfast and one other meal. Even 'fully' catered halls do not necessarily provide three meals seven days a week; investigate this when budgeting for food. Catered halls may use pre-paid card systems that reward you with food at a reduced price. Dietary requirements can usually be catered for if advance warning is given. Good-sized kitchens are supplied for self-catered halls. Even catered halls provide a small kitchen for making snacks and drinks. *Warning*: catered halls often have short mealtimes. Medical courses often require you to be out a lot more than other courses. Find out the feasibility of getting to your hall in time for meals if you choose a catered hall; otherwise you may pay for a service which is impossible to use.

➡ *En suite rooms or shared bathroom facilities*: *en suite* halls are generally more expensive, but preferred by those who do not want to have to queue for a shower or be seen before they are fully dressed. Some halls with shared bathroom facilities provide a sink in each room.

➡ *Undergraduate or postgraduate*: universities try to place postgraduates with postgraduates and undergraduates with undergraduates – as a result some halls only cater for one of these groups.

➡ *Mixed or single-sex*: Single-sex halls of residence exist. If this is your preference, consult the accommodation information for details.

Facilities

The facilities provided by halls differ; however, most offer the following.

➡ *Telephones*: calls are usually free within the university and university residences, but external calls and external incoming calls are often expensive.

➡ *Internet*: various options for internet are now available, including broadband connections in each room and wireless connections. Services may be free (e.g. for wireless), or carry a cost as an initial subscription or a per-minute-rate.

➡ *Laundry*: there is often a laundry associated with the halls; however, these usually involve a charge per wash.

Some facilities may have added extras, look out for:

➡ café, restaurant or bar – not just in catered halls
➡ games and/or television room
➡ computer and/or library area
➡ music practice rooms
➡ sports facilities

➥ health advice centre
➥ cash machine.

Advantages of living in halls

Halls provide a quick and easy way of making new friends. The majority of students are away from home and know few people. Where better to make friends than over a cup of tea in your shared living room?

Only students live in halls, so there is usually someone with whom you can travel to university or get a taxi home after a night out. Events within halls may be organised by the social or hall committee such as welcoming events, balls, parties and trips. Although a small fee may be requested, any profit is usually spent on improving the hall services.

Often bills are included in the cost of hall accommodation. With so many things to think about when you leave home for the first time, this is one less thing to worry about.

Halls usually have wardens / sub-wardens / resident assistants available 24 hours a day. These individuals are responsible for welfare and discipline. They ensure you always have support if you encounter problems. In addition, some halls employ security guards. This increases your safety in comparison to private accommodation.

Disadvantages of living in halls

Distractions are rife in halls. You can usually hear exactly what is going on in the room next door. Fireproof doors are everywhere and always bang shut; an unwelcome noise at four in the morning. Some students love to set off fire alarms in the middle of the night . . . every night. Usually in your first year work stress levels are low enough to cope with this, but when final exams are looming, avoiding such disruption can be important.

Hall rooms are often small and poorly furnished. Usually they can be quickly decorated and personalised (providing you do not contravene rules regarding sticking things to walls, etc.); however, the initial impression of a grotty room can remain with you for a good while.

Often hall contracts do not include holidays. This can result in tediously regular moves every holiday. You may feel unsettled and your belongings may get damaged through regular packing, unpacking and moving.

Depending on the standard of your halls, they can be expensive. Previous residents may have clearly left their mark. More expensive halls may be *en suite* or recently renovated, but do not expect money to buy you space.

Other university accommodation

Some universities own accommodation apart from halls, or have partnerships with local landlords. These can be a good alternative to halls as the accommodation is more closely regulated than private accommodation. However, competition for this accommodation is high and you may be in limbo until close to term time while you wait for news of an allocation. This option may be more expensive than similar, private properties; however, you are paying for quality assurance and support if problems occur.

Home

If you are attending a medical school near to your family home you may choose to stay there. This can be great if your family encourages you to work and to rest in appropriate proportions. Meals may be cooked for you and it may be a cheaper option. However, demands from family, friends and/or dependents may distract you from your study. You may feel excluded from the student lifestyle and may be a distance from regular student haunts. If you are in a position to live at home, still consider your other accommodation options, especially if finances are not a restraint.

Private accommodation

You may rent private accommodation alone or with friends. The latter may be difficult in the first year if you do not know anyone else in the university. Living alone may also become isolating.

Private accommodation can provide support if you are living with friends. There will always be someone you know and like on hand if you need a shoulder to cry on or a ready source of entertainment. If you are living with other medical students you will have live-in study partners. The quality of private accommodation usually varies consistently with price.

Drawbacks to private accommodation occur if you realise you and your flatmates are not such good friends after all. Space suddenly disappears and privacy goes out the window. Exam times can be stressful if you are all medical students and this can make relaxation difficult. Conversely, study can be difficult as a result of regular social distractions. Student accommodation is often a target for burglars, especially when holidays are long and your belongings are left in the accommodation; but do not be falsely reassured, student accommodation also gets burgled during term time. Finally, choices for private accommodation may be limited for students and minimum contracts are often longer than you require; you often have to rent for 12 months when you only need nine.

Own house

It was while looking at rental properties for my second year at medical school that my family decided to buy a house rather than rent. Since I was going to be living in the same place for at least four years it made sense for the money otherwise spent on renting to go towards a mortgage. If we could get people to rent the other rooms then all the better. I have now just finished my course, and looking back at my time as a live-in landlady, it has definitely been worthwhile financially, but is not without problems.

The first obvious advantage of this kind of investment is the potential to make money during your time at university. The length of the course should give you time to recoup some of the money put into buying and furnishing the property. However, a profit is not guaranteed and you could end up with an overall loss. Availability of willing tenants is uncertain – you may think you have plenty of friends who would like to rent from you, but four years is a long time, situations change and people move around. You have to be prepared to find new tenants each year and live with people you do not know in order to fill your rooms.

The possibility that you might have to move also needs to be considered. Many medical schools operate in hospitals some miles from the main campus. Find out if you will be expected to do placements in other towns and for how long. The recent changes in job applications also mean that you may have/want to move once you qualify.

Most of the time being a live-in landlady has been no different than just living in a normal shared house. However, you do feel the pressure to find tenants who will look after your property, which can be difficult. You also have to take more responsibility for the property. If the boiler breaks or a tap needs fixing, your housemates will be looking to you to sort it out. As a medical student you already have quite a lot on your plate and, on occasion, the last thing you need to be worrying about is a house or tenant on top of all that. Finally, you may sometimes feel restricted. I would have loved to live on my own in my final year, but I had to rent the rooms to cover the mortgage.

All in all, I am glad my family owned a house while I was at university, but I would urge anyone considering it to think very carefully. (*Catherine Taylor, fifth-year medical student, Manchester*)

Owning property is not an option for many students. Money is tight and buying a house is way down the agenda. In many circumstances when a house is bought for university, the parents buy the house (and put it in the student's name) and the student lives in it as a live-in landlord/landlady. There are many advantages to (you or your family) owning the house you live in during university:

➡ you will not have to move in and out for holiday periods
➡ you will not have to look for new accommodation each year
➡ you know the quality of your accommodation
➡ you can have more control over whom you live with
➡ you are on the housing ladder before you graduate
➡ your course is long; owning your house will prevent expenditure on rent with no returns.

However, there are some disadvantages to owning a house:
➡ it can be lonely if you live by yourself
➡ you may get frustrated/upset if housemates do not care for the house as you wish them to
➡ you have a responsibility to fix things as they break
➡ unexpected costs can become unmanageable on tight student budgets
➡ you may face long commutes or periods in which your house is empty if your placements are a long way away.

If you/your family are considering buying a house for your student years, first investigate the following.
➡ Where are your clinical placements at medical school likely to be?
➡ What junior doctor jobs are available in the area?
➡ Different mortgage options, e.g. all-in-one accounts that combine your mortgage and current account, provide great flexibility in paying back the mortgage. They allow minimal payments while you are a student but also allow an unlimited increase in payments as your salary rises during your career. These mortgages provide you with the opportunity to pay off your mortgage much sooner than with fixed payment mortgages. Depending on your circumstances, parents or a partner may be required to qualify for a mortgage.

Accommodation during clinical placements

If your clinical placements are not within a reasonably commutable distance, your medical school has some responsibilities for your accommodation. You should not pay for two residences. Familiarity with the appropriate standards (*see* Appendix IV) will ensure your medical school provides you with appropriate accommodation options. The standards are designed to prevent you from travelling long distances when you are tired and to utilise your time with study, rather than travel.[1]

> Wherever you live during university (term time and holidays), write down the address and keep it safe. You will require your previous five-year address history whenever you change hospitals/trusts/jobs, etc. for your Criminal Record Bureau (or equivalent) checks.

Some final considerations

If all that was not enough to think about, there are a few more considerations to make.
➡ *Crockery, cutlery and cooking utensils* – supplied?
➡ *Bedding and towels* – supplied? If they are supplied, are they washed?
➡ *Bills* – included or not? If so, which ones? If not, how much are they?

➨ *Additional needs* – for example, do you need wheelchair access or accommodation that allows a guide dog? Get in contact with the Student Accommodation Office or your university's Disability Office.

➨ *Cleaning* – is a cleaner employed to clean your halls? Beware, cleaners will only clean up if they can see the surfaces they are supposed to be cleaning (i.e. be tidy).

➨ *Contract terms* – the cost, number of weeks, payment schedule and accommodation during holidays. Remember that academic years for medical students can be longer than for other students.

➨ *Route to university* –safe? Far? University transport? Remember clinical placements do not occur in university buildings.

➨ *Parking* – can you bring your car (you often cannot at halls)? Is a permit required? Are there facilities to safely store your bicycle?

➨ *Content insurance* – included or not? If not, get some.

➨ *Furniture* – what? Halls usually provide a bed, desk, chair, wardrobe, chest of drawers and some shelves – anything else you need?

HOW TO COPE WITH LIVING AWAY FROM HOME

Cooking

You may go to university having never cooked before or you may have accomplished skills. However, cooking on a budget, often in confined spaces within university accommodation, with limited storage space and minimal cooking equipment will stretch even the most capable cooks. One solution is to live in catered halls. However, this may not be possible, especially after your first year. So how do you keep yourself well nourished during university?

Medicine is mentally and physically demanding. Eat well to feed your mind and body but also make things that are quick and easy. Think about the types of food you enjoy which are healthy, cheap and easy to cook. Examples of such recipes can be found below in Boxes 12.1, 12.2 and 12.3.

Everyone is advised to take five portions of fruit and vegetables each day as part of a healthy diet. Such portions include raw, cooked, frozen and canned food. Unfortunately, fresh fruit and vegetables are often not as cheap, per meal, as the frozen pizzas in the next aisle. Supermarkets are addressing this by introducing fruit and vegetables to value ranges. Supermarkets sell fruit and vegetables both pre-packed and loose; the loose produce is usually cheapest. Another way of buying cheap fruit and vegetables is on a market stall. Some universities have fruit and vegetable trailers/shops, so look out for these.

Ways to improve your fruit and vegetable intake without breaking the bank can include:

➨ snack on carrot sticks instead of crisps

➨ add tinned/frozen vegetables to rice/pasta

➥ add a banana to breakfast cereal
➥ buy value range fruit juice and substitute one non-juice drink a day with this.

A good starting point for any student, other than the designated 'student cookbooks' (which often contain cheap but unhealthy food), is the food goddess herself, Delia Smith. No house is complete without the *Complete Illustrated Cookery Course*.[2] This book contains recipes for basic foods, including simple explanations of useful cooking techniques and conversion charts.

Box 12.1 Recipe for tomato sauce

If you like it, you will soon discover what a fantastic source of food and nutrition pasta can be. It is cheap, some can be cooked in less than five minutes and it is versatile. The following is a vague recipe, on the basis that you may not have kitchen scales, to give you the basis of many a meal: a vegetable and tomato sauce. Depending on what you put in, this will be enough for two to four servings.

Ingredients
1–2 onions, chopped
1 tablespoon oil – vegetable, sunflower or olive – olive oil is best but the most expensive, vegetable oil is the cheapest
Vegetable stock cube (optional) – adds flavour
2 teaspoons mixed herbs – often in value ranges and make a plain meal much more tasty
Tin of tomatoes – value range tins are absolutely fine (often costing less than 20p)
Half-tube of tomato purée – makes the sauce richer
Vegetables – roughly chopped to similar sizes (mushrooms, carrots, courgettes, peppers, aubergines, leeks, etc.)
Pasta – one or two handfuls per person
Cheese – (cheddar or parmesan) grated to put on the top; cheddar cheese can often be found in value ranges
Black pepper – to taste

Method
Put the chopped onion in a pan over a medium heat, oil is not required if using a non-stick pan. Make sure you stir the onions well to stop them sticking. Cook until they have become a bit more 'see-through'. At this stage you can add the herbs, black pepper and stock cube (but, beware, the onions stick more easily once the stock cube has been added to the pan). Add any vegetables you have chopped and stir these until they have softened slightly. Add the tin of tomatoes and the tomato purée. Bring the sauce to the boil and then reduce the heat under the pan and let the sauce bubble gently (simmering) until it has thickened; this usually takes about five minutes, but make sure you keep stirring it. You can always add

---

Box 12.1 cont.

water if the sauce gets too thick. While the sauce is simmering you can cook the pasta according to the instructions on the packet. Once the pasta is cooked (you can test this by trying a piece) strain out the water and add the pasta to your sauce. If the sauce is still too thin cook it for a little longer, otherwise the meal is ready to serve. Put it into a bowl and sprinkle a little grated cheese on the top.

If you are cooking for one, you can still make the above quantity – it keeps in the fridge for two to three days really well and the flavours increase as it sits there. You can then re-heat the meal in a pan or a microwave. It also freezes very well, but you may not want to add the pasta to the sauce before freezing it.

Variations

Meaty pasta – cook some lean minced beef, diced chicken breast or chopped bacon with the onions at the beginning of the recipe; once this is cooked through add the vegetables and tomato and continue as before.

Vegetarian pasta – you may want a bit more substance or protein; just add a tin of cooked kidney beans, butter beans or lentils when you add the tinned tomatoes. You can also use the meaty pasta variation, but make it with meat substitutes such as Quorn, which can be like chicken or minced beef.

Posh pasta – you may be trying to impress a new love interest, show your parents your culinary skills or just want to treat yourself. Add chopped bacon to the onions, then some chopped olives, sun-dried tomatoes and a glass of red wine (you can have fun researching good, cheap wine). Try adding a teaspoon of pesto as well.

Pasta bake – using any of the above variations, mix the pasta with the sauce, place it in an ovenproof dish and sprinkle grated cheese and a slice of grated bread on the top, then bake in the oven at a high heat for 10–15 minutes, or until crisp.

Student risotto – at the stage when you have just finished cooking the vegetables and are about to add the tinned tomatoes add a couple of handfuls of rice for each person. Then add the tinned tomatoes and about a can of water. You may also want to add another stock cube. Cook this for about half an hour until the rice is tender, stirring frequently and adding more water as required.

Pizza – reduce the sauce until it is really thick, with very little juice, spoon the mixture onto a ready-made pizza base and sprinkle some cheese over it. Hey presto! A healthy pizza.

Box 12.2 Recipe for white sauce

White or cheese sauce can be mixed with macaroni, topped with cheese and put under the grill (macaroni cheese), poured over cooked broccoli and/or cauliflower (broccoliflower cheese!) or layered with the meaty tomato sauce from Box 12.1 and sheets of pasta to make lasagne. You will have to experiment with the recipe

Box 12.2 cont.
below to make the quantity you need if you do not have kitchen scales or a measuring jug.

Ingredients
Knob of butter
Plain flour
Milk
Handful of grated cheese (for cheese sauce)

Method
Place the knob of butter in a pan over a low heat and stir until it is melted. Add the flour and blend with the melted butter until you end up with a mixture resembling wet breadcrumbs. Add some milk, a bit at a time, mixing well each time until your sauce is thick, smooth and runny. Add the cheese (for the cheese sauce), stir until it has melted and your sauce is ready.

Box 12.3 Recipe for omelette
An omelette is a quick, easy, nutritious and healthy meal to rustle up. You may have it as an entire meal, or a plain omelette can be cut into strips and laid over a pasta or rice dish instead of cheese.

Ingredients
1–3 eggs per serving
Splash of milk
Knob of butter or margarine
Filling (onion, bacon, mushrooms, peppers, cheese)

Method
Whisk (using a fork if you don't have a whisk) the eggs with a splash of milk until mixed thoroughly and the mixture is a bit frothy. Place the knob of butter/ margarine in a frying pan over a low heat and stir until it has melted. Add the egg and milk mixture to the pan and stir it around in the pan until it starts to set (it looks a bit like scrambled egg for a few seconds). Once the egg mixture is really setting, and has covered the entire base of the frying pan, leave it to cook. If you are using a filling, add this to your omelette now. Wait until it is cooked through, then fold your omelette in half and serve with salad, vegetables or baked beans.

Kitchen equipment you will need

The kitchen equipment you require depends on the accommodation you have. Information on the equipment provided is published in the university accommodation pack. As a general rule:

➡ *Catered halls*: you will require equipment to make snacks and drinks; however, a kettle will usually be provided.
➡ *Self-catered halls*: a kettle, microwave, fridge/freezer, toaster and cooker are usually provided.
➡ *University/rented accommodation*: depends on your contract but a fridge/freezer, cooker and kettle and/or microwave are often provided.
➡ *Private accommodation*: this varies with every property.

Storage space in hall and rented, shared accommodation is usually reduced to one cupboard and one fridge shelf each. Remember this when buying equipment to take with you. The excess will need to be stored in your bedroom.

Equipment to consider taking may include the following.
➡ *Drinks and snacks*: mugs, plates and bowls (two of each), cutlery, sharp knife, storage boxes, sandwich toaster (optional but common!).
➡ *Cooking*: chopping board, potato peeler, pans (two or three), heatproof spoon and spatula, potato masher, whisk, oven gloves, scissors, cheese grater, oven proof dish (e.g. glass dishes with lids), mixing bowls, clingfilm, foil.
➡ *Washing up*: tea towels, washing up cloths/brush/scourer.

Some companies sell starter kits with students in mind, for example The Cooks Kitchen (http://thecookskitchen.com/browse_8894). Even if you do not need the whole set you can look at these for ideas.

Food-shopping

Only go food-shopping once a week. This provides plenty of fresh food but reduces time wasted by going too often. In addition, if you go more often you will probably end up buying more than you need, as you may be tempted by offers and impulse buys.

Find out which supermarkets are closest to your accommodation. You may notice significant differences in price between companies so shop around. Avoid shopping in convenience stores because they tend to be more expensive. Many supermarkets have loyalty or reward cards. It is worth taking advantage of these, as they are free and points soon add up to significant rewards.

Buy food from the value ranges. Basic store-cupboard ingredients such as tinned tomatoes, flour, cheese and pasta can all be found in value ranges.

Make a list of what you need. Think about the basic foods you consume daily, roughly plan your meals for the week and then allow yourself a few extras. You may not have money to throw around and shopping without a list can be expensive if you buy too much. Box 12.4 offers a basic template from which you can build your shopping list.

> **Box 12.4 Template shopping list**
>
> | | |
> |---|---|
> | Milk | Margarine/butter |
> | Bread | Cheese |
> | Cereal, porridge | Tea, coffee, hot chocolate, etc. |
> | Sugar | Pasta |
> | Vegetables | Tinned vegetables, soups, beans or fish |
> | Fruit | Lunch box items (yoghurts, crisps, biscuits) |
> | Meat | Rice |
> | Jam, marmalade, honey, etc. | Eggs |
> | Sandwich fillings | Flour |

MEDICAL STUDENTS AND CARS

Unfortunately many medical students feel they require a car at some point. This is an important problem, as cars represent a huge expense. In a culture of widening participation it is obscene that students have to consider the need for driving lessons let alone buying/running a car.

Financially, the considerations include payments of:

➡ finance (if applicable)
➡ fuel
➡ insurance (on-road parking increases costs)
➡ tax
➡ roadside rescue cover
➡ servicing and MOT
➡ car-parking costs or permits
➡ repairs.

Students living in halls may have parking banned or restricted on the grounds of the accommodation and thus have to park a reasonable distance away to avoid being clamped or fined.

Medical students can usually manage without a car in their pre-clinical years. Indeed, parking around universities and hospitals is notoriously difficult and best avoided. Most UK medical schools are based in or around major towns and cities which have well-developed, regular, reliable and easily accessed public transport. Although costs vary with location, week/month/year passes often minimise expense. You will usually be able to access route maps, timetables and fare charge information for local bus, tram and train companies online.

Food shopping can be awkward without a car but alternatives include:

➡ Courtesy buses associated with halls and/or specific supermarkets
➡ Internet shopping: even without splitting delivery costs between flatmates this will work out cheaper than buying a car just to get you to the shops.

Placements can be difficult to reach (safely) by public transport; a car is a preferred option in these cases. Often, universities try to identify the students who have cars and allocate these students to placements that are tricky to reach using public transport. Even if public transport is available, it can take up a large amount of time; a half-hour car journey may equate to a two-hour bus journey. In addition, some placements are located in areas in which it would be unsafe to wait for public transport to arrive. However, some areas are not safe to leave a car. Speak to your tutors, previous students and people at your placement for local information.

Decide on your personal financial priorities when contemplating buying a car. Many medical students get through their entire degree without being able to drive, some wait until their clinical placements to buy a car and others have a car from the start – whatever you decide you won't be alone.

SOCIETIES, CLUBS AND ACTIVITY GROUPS

University provides opportunity to join societies, clubs and activity groups; recreational, international, departmental, academic, cultural (arts, music, performance), religious or political. However, if the university-based groups are not for you, or you want to embrace your local community, community groups also exist. If the society you desire does not exist, start your own. Try to follow your interests as they provide a reason to have a rest from work and provide interest on your future job application forms.

Joining societies, clubs or activity groups is a good way of meeting like-minded people and getting an introduction to the local area.

Information on the available societies, clubs and groups at each university can be found in prospectuses and institution websites.

SPORT

If you are serious about sport, university clubs and teams are numerous. There are university teams for most sports and medical school teams for many. You can enter a team or club at any level from beginner to elite or professional, or you can get involved in coaching or organising the team and events. Do not be scared to investigate what is on offer at your university – something will suit your desires.

University or medical school clubs are often competitive. If all you want to do is have a weekly game or kick-around, arrange a friendly game among your peers. University sports facilities are usually cheap to hire. Medical defence organisations sometimes offer money to spend on team kits/bibs. Ask your local representative about this.

CULTURE AND RELAXATION

Universities and cities have a wealth of culture and entertainment. If you enjoy the cinema, look out for one on your university campus. Otherwise, local cinemas often have student discounts.

Universities often have their own art galleries, museums and theatres. Information on exhibitions and other local cultural attractions will be available from the university and local tourist information.

You may have considered the local shops when you chose which medical schools to apply to. Shopping can be a great way of getting away from your study and treating yourself after some hard work. Do not forget, many high street shops offer student discounts to National Union of Student (NUS) cardholders; make sure you carry this valuable card on all shopping trips.

Do not forget, you can enjoy culture and relax on your own with a good novel.

> Have non-medic friends and keep in touch with people from home. It's good to keep grounded and have a good support network. (*Rachel Boyce, third-year medical student, Aberdeen*)

SOCIALISING

With all the new people you meet at medical school and university you are bound to be doing lots of socialising. This may revolve around pubs, bars or clubs or you may have friends with whom you undertake interests or just stay in with and watch films or TV. Whatever you do, socialising is important. You need your friends around you when the going gets tough, but more importantly, you need friends around you to prevent the going getting tough.

Do not forget those friends you have left behind. Your old friends may know you better than anyone, you will really regret it if you let them slip. It is easy for a whole term to pass and realise you have not been in contact with the person who you used to spend every evening with. Make regular arrangements to meet up or arrange to call them every week on a particular day; you will remain in contact and keep up with all the gossip from home.

> Medicine is a vocation and it requires a lot of your time and energy. You have to give a part of your life to medicine, and in order to do this you must have something to give in the first place. Having a life away from work also maintains your sanity, keeps your feet on the ground and provides you with the skills you need to talk to patients. It is very easy to make excuses to get out of socialising if you have work to do; however, if you socialise regularly your people skills will be a lot better. Remember that doctors and patients are both human. The only difference is that one has a few clinical skills and a bit more medical knowledge than the other – that's all. (*Paul White, second-year medical student, St Andrews*)

It is great to spend time with medics, but make sure you have non-medic friends as well. *(Nat Bradbrook, fifth-year medical student, Manchester)*

Student Union

Socialising at university often centres on the Student Union. You are an automatic member of your university's Student Union. The Student Union is a building and a concept. As a building, it often houses single or multiple cafes, bars, clubs, shops, offices and society headquarters. There is also often a large hall that houses a wide variety of events from career fairs to rock concerts. Other features may include cinemas, printing services, travel agents, Post Offices, markets, beauty parlours, laundrettes, radio stations or student newspapers. The concept of the Student Union is that it provides students with the support and services they require. As a result, Student Unions contain information on study, finances, jobs, health and sexuality as well as a student advice centre. The Student Union also represents the voice of the student body, through lobbying of the university and/or Government.

Student Unions are designed for use on a 24 hour basis. You can buy your breakfast (cheap) there before you start the day, grab a bite for lunch and pick up some stationery, get a drink at the end of the day (very cheap) and go out clubbing in the evening. The Student Union is there for you so use it to the full.

Information on the Student Union at each university is provided in the respective prospectuses and on their websites.

INTIMATE RELATIONSHIPS[3]

You will all have friendships, some within and outside of the medical community. However, medicine does not leave much time for forming intimate relationships. After all, romance is lost when you have to take an anatomy textbook to an expensive restaurant because you have an exam the next day. Single, senior medical students and junior doctors often despair at the lack of 'talent' in their hospital and long for a boozy night out to a club to meet the local 'hot stuff'. They then meet with the realisation that work, study and existing friendships are already taking up all their time. But do not despair, many medical students find and keep a partner and some get married while at medical school. So what are the problems and the benefits of finding, forming and keeping intimate relationships as a medical student (and professional)?

Benefits of having an intimate partner

A happy relationship will often result in a happy you. It is reassuring to know that if you have a bad day, you will go home to someone who cares about and loves you.

Those of you who have partnered with non-medical individuals will be able to relish non-medical conversation and an uncompetitive home environment. Exam stress is not heightened by there being two nervous wrecks trying to support each other. Indeed, the fact that you have a partner who is not involved with your exams may enable you to put things into perspective and not let stress ruin your mental and physical health. You may greatly benefit each other by using the experiences gained from different workplaces to advise on problems. Conversely, if you are involved with a medic, you will have somebody whom you can ask for a fully informed second opinion, as they will understand many of the problems you may have, they will appreciate the stress that exams bring and they will know the problems that are unique to training in the medical profession.

If you are involved with another medic, they will understand the pressures you face. Partners look out for each other. You are going to be under pressure throughout your life. Often, your partner knows you better than anyone and will be able to promptly detect the signs that you are not coping. This will encourage you to seek help before you reach crisis point.

What can go wrong with medical professionals' intimate relationships?

Despite the benefits, for those of you who have partnered up with non-medical individuals, it may not always be plain sailing. Your partner may not fully understand (despite how often you tell them) how much pressure you are under and how much work you have to do. Working long hours or nights can result in your partner feeling neglected or second-best.

If your relationship is with another medic, it may be difficult to avoid medical talk. Automatic limitations are imposed if your partner has minimal knowledge on diseases; however, if you both are experts and enthusiasts you will accidentally slip into work talk in private time. Private time itself may be limited in a medic–medic relationship, as you will both have work pressures, long hours and periods of exhaustion. The resulting lack of relaxing time together can put great strain on even the best partnerships.

If you have a medical partner you may find yourself undertaking competitive job applications that may result in offers of jobs in totally different geographical locations. You must make the decision to live apart for some time or for one of you to embark on a career in a less competitive specialty in order to get jobs in the same area. Some consideration is given for linked applications to some jobs; however, allocations for linked jobs are based on the weaker of the two applicants.

Giving your relationship the best chance for survival

Do not leave 'couple-time' to arrange itself: aim to have one meal together each day and ban medical topics. Your timetable, study or work can be erratic, so pre-allocate some time during the week for you to spend together and keep this time free. Once your time together is secured, take full advantage of it. Go out and away from books, telephones and emails. Undertake hobbies or activities together. Try playing sport, doing the gardening or cooking a special meal?

Make time to see your non-medical friends and family. Do not just let your social lives revolve around 'medic's do's'. Discuss your priorities. Whether you are both medics or not, you will both have priorities. You need to make sure you both know the others' priorities early in the relationship to avoid conflict in the future. If your priorities do not match, reach a compromise that you both agree with.

Think about your ideal future careers. Which of you is going to be more flexible to allow the other to move for more sought-after jobs? Who can take time off work if you decide to have children? If neither of you can, or want to be, flexible, make sure you have an acceptable contingency plan set in your minds as early as possible so you are not faced with difficult, unexpected problems.

STUDENTS WITH FAMILIES, CHILDREN AND/OR DEPENDANTS

With graduate-entry courses and mature medical students being increasingly encouraged, the issue of medical students with families, children and/or dependants becomes more important. Support from academic staff and sympathetic placement allocation are often perceived as good. However, some students do not feel they are aware of all their options. So what is available for medical students with families, children and/or dependants?[4]

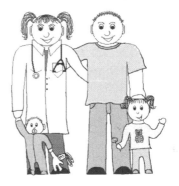

The most common form of support from medical schools for medical students with children or dependants is financial (*see* Chapter 11). However, support may also involve the following.[5]

Childcare

Free or subsidised childcare provision for medical students has been proposed, but this may not be in place during your time at medical school. Investigate all childcare options. Some universities and/or student unions offer nursery places. However, competition for places is high and they can be costly. Before you register your child in a university nursery find out about holiday opening; your terms often run into the normal university holidays. Be clear about the ages of children the childcare allows as this varies between universities. If your university does not provide childcare, or if it is full, they may be able to give you details of nurseries, childminders and after school services. Further sources of information on childcare options can be found in the care arrangements section of www.support4doctors.org and at www.childcarelink.gov.uk.

Practical support

If you have children or dependants you should be able to request clinical placements near your home, if available. Some universities also run schemes that allow you to hire safety items for children (e.g. fireguards, stair gates and cots) for a small charge.

Emotional support

Individual universities may have contacts or groups for student parents. Use these contacts as they may provide helpful advice, support and information. Contact existing students with dependants before applying to medical school to gain an understanding of the level of support available. Contact the university for details of how to do this.

Maternity leave

If you expect to become pregnant during your student years, contact your prospective universities/medical schools to find out about their maternity leave policies. If you are an existing student planning a pregnancy try and gain all the information you can before falling pregnant. If your pregnancy is unexpected, inform your medical school of your pregnancy as early as you can and you will be able to make plans for the maternity period.

FURTHER READING

www.funky.co.uk (UK online student community)

Houghton A. Personal support 3: how to help someone achieve balance in their working and personal lives. *BMJ Career Focus.* 2005; **331**: 7–8.

www.medical-student.co.uk (Website for a UK wide, free medical student publication)

Medics on the move (www.medicsonthemove.co.uk) (National relocation and home search service for medics, lawyers, accountants and all busy professionals)

CHAPTER 13

Medical student socials

Medical students are renowned for consumption of large volumes of alcohol. So what might you expect from a medical student social?

⏩ **Who needs a reason? . . . let's just go out.**

You are out for an evening with a group of people you know. Staggering into your sixteenth pub, boys wearing nothing but a flimsy nighty and girls wearing cute slippers, you all suddenly stop. Everyone has simultaneously recognised one of the group leaving a fast-food outlet with a burger. A familiar condemnation ensues 'eating is cheating'. Where are you? A medical student social.

Medical student socials epitomise everything you are learning not to do. Drinking copious amounts of alcohol, smoking and eating greasy food (if you can get away with it). Medical students enjoy a good night out. Indeed, good days out come a close second; day trips to theme parks are not uncommon. Medical students 'let their hair down' regularly, and who can blame them? Carefree, fun nights are a welcome contrast to the hard slog of university. Some medical students will be socialising most nights. Year groups are often so large that subsections will be continually organising something. Specific events that are often 'celebrated' are medical student birthdays, end of exams/terms, start of terms, Halloween, Easter, Christmas and exam results.

You work all day together. So why do medical students also socialise with other medical students?

➡ medical students may be the only people you know in an area, especially if your medical school or placement is separate from the main university
➡ work hard – play hard
➡ exams at the same time
➡ every year counts; everyone understands the others' pressures
➡ large numbers of medical students ensure a good turnout at social events.

It's great to be involved with medics' activities, but do not limit yourself solely to these. Medical schools thrive on gossip. Having another set of friends or activities will partially detach you from this. *(Zoe Cowan, first-year medical student, Leicester)*

What are the disadvantages of medical student socials?
➡ There will be nowhere to hide. Do not do anything you may regret, you will be working with the witnesses everyday.
➡ You may get sick of each other. Usually, people only rarely go out with colleagues.
➡ If you do not want to go out it can be very difficult to say no. Feelings of exclusion occur when everyone is talking about the night before, the next day.
➡ Medical student socials are frequent and often mid-week. This may affect your study in and out of university.

FUND-RAISING

Medical students are resourceful when giving to their local community. Fund-raising is an excuse for even more crazy behaviour during socials. Funds are raised for charities, the medical school and medical student groups.

Fund-raising ideas are broad and may include the following.
➡ *Slave auctions*: medical students and their assets are auctioned and sold to the highest bidder.
➡ *Sponsored walks, bike rides, swims, etc.*: this alone may not be crazy enough for medical students so doing it in fancy dress is preferred and racks up the pounds.
➡ *Themed pub-crawls*: fancy dress (scrubs, pyjamas), three-legged.
➡ *Balls*: Christmas, graduation, Freshers, end of year . . .
➡ *Parties or discos*: often held at local clubs and true to form they are often themed . . . Halloween, Valentine's, Christmas, back-to-school, tarts and vicars, you name it, it has probably been done.
➡ *Plays*: based upon a known story or devised from scratch, medical student plays usually incorporate jokes about notorious tutors, lecturers and students.
➡ *Fashion shows*.
➡ Those who are not faint-hearted may even undertake skydives, bungee jumping and abseiling.

CHAPTER 14

When things go wrong

Go ahead and take risks. Just be sure that everything will turn out ok.[1]

Perhaps a surprise that this chapter is not entitled 'If things go wrong', but this would be falsely optimistic. Medical school is tough. There will be times for everyone when things go wrong. Read on for advice on some of the more common problems that you may face while at medical school.

BAD DAYS

What constitutes a bad day? A patient dying? Feeling like you have learnt nothing? Getting home too late to watch your favourite television programme? Learn to recognise what has made you feel like you have had a bad day then identify ways of improving your mood and preventing it happening again. You cannot plan for every bad day; however, support from friends and family, hobbies and learning the concepts of professionalism will certainly help.

> The big surprise has been friends. The term has been made much more enjoyable and my learning better by getting to know people and learning with them in groups, especially dissection and anatomy. It makes me feel better to know that I am not alone. (*Pauline Law, first-year medical student, Dundee*)

Common situations and possible solutions
Staff

Sometimes staff members do not want you around, at other times you do not want to be working; both can result in you upsetting the staff. Sort out problems as they arise to improve the 'atmosphere', yours and their piece of mind and your educational progress. Hospitals, GP surgeries and medical schools are intimately related. Any distaste towards you from staff will quickly get around. Swallow your pride and act quickly to enable your side of the situation to be considered.

Tutors

Your tutors want to assist your education. If they are giving you a hard time, ask yourself 'Is their behaviour appropriate?' You may feel 'picked on' when really you just got frustrated because you could not answer questions or you felt silly when you failed at a skill. If this is the case, learn the answers/skill/etc., and move on.

Peers

You will not always get on with your peers and an easy solution to this is not always possible. Avoid those people you have issues with, whilst remaining professional. Focus on something positive that is going to happen after the group/encounter is over. Be courteous, polite and communicate required information at all times; otherwise you may become someone else's issue.

Life can be a battle

As a medical student and doctor you face many battles; for example, against patients 'informed' by the internet, against nursing staff who 'know about medical students' and peers who want to undermine you. Detect the early warning signs that battle is about to commence, then strategically avoid it and prospectively manage the situation. If all else fails, calmly explain your position and leave. Battles cannot always be won, but they cannot be lost if they do not begin.

Feeling useless

Sometimes you feel you have no particular role within the team or group in which you are working. This makes you feel useless and undermines your self-confidence. Ask if you can have a regular job or responsibility, for example collecting investigation results; this will also free up time for your colleagues to teach you. Problem-based learning enables all members of the learning group to have a role, rotating on a weekly basis; make sure this happens.

> Students may have to work in a group whereby you may have the misfortune of being placed with people that you do not like, or do not get along with. I find it really emotionally draining. I came to medicine with an open mind and with great enthusiasm. While I find the study and clinical training really enjoyable, I have found working within a group of eight students, day-in, day-out . . . particularly hard. (*Anonymous*)

Just a bad day

Sometimes days are just bad. You may be under the weather, feeling tired or just not in the mood for university. These days happen to the best of people. Start tomorrow afresh.

FAILING EXAMS

> It's not just teaching staff who suddenly disappear when asked for help by failing students; colleagues and friends do, too . . . it's not that friends don't want to help, it's just that they don't know what to say or do, and failing students aren't keen to seek help from their more successful colleagues.[2]

The General Medical Council (GMC) states that 'only those students who are fit to practice as doctors should be allowed to complete the curriculum and gain provisional registration'.[3] Exams are designed to assess your competency and fitness to practice. Those who are not up to standard should fail. However, failing exams may not just be due to incompetence. Pass thresholds for medical school exams are often based upon mean scores and standard deviations of your cohort. Thus a certain proportion of medical students will fail each time. You may fail because your marks were comparatively lower than the other people in your year, not because you do not know anything. Poor exam technique, extreme nerves, illness, personal issues, poor preparation or lack of information on the content or structure of the exam can also lead to failure. Disclose any problems you have, that you think may affect your academic progress, as soon as possible. Confidentiality will be maintained (unless you represent a danger to others).

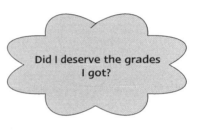

Did I deserve the grades I got?

Each medical school will have a Progress Committee, or similar group. This group will call to see you if you fail exams, re-sits or there is concern about your academic performance from those involved in your training. The Progress Committee will provide you with options should you fail your exams. It is thus important that your academic and personal records are good and 'clean' otherwise your fail will not be looked upon favourably and your options may be reduced.

If you have a good past record and there is a good explanation for your recent fail, complete failure may not occur in all cases. Your average mark may be worked out to cancel one failed exam. In this case you will pass overall. If your fail mark was close to a pass, you may be invited to take a pass/fail viva (oral exam). If you have failed a number of exams or have given the committee cause for concern you may be required to re-sit the year. Dropping

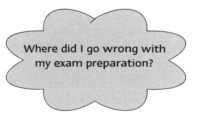

Where did I go wrong with my exam preparation?

out of medical school is unlikely to be a first choice option in most cases. However, if you have set a pattern of failing, you have given your university cause for concern for other reasons (e.g. conduct) or you really do not have any motivation this may be the best or most appropriate option.

If you have to re-sit an exam, seek support from your medical school who will often offer help with revision. They may provide access to skills laboratories or tutoring. In your clinical years, local doctors may take you under their wing if they know you are struggling but believe in your practical abilities. Do not lose hope. Take all options available to you and get your head down to study.

DROPPING OUT OF MEDICAL SCHOOL

Some medical students drop out of medical school because they realise it is 'not for them'. Any amount of prior experience will not fully prepare you for what medical school and a medical career entails. The hard work, rapid maturation, devastating experiences and unpleasant people you meet along the way may not balance the fantastic experiences available to you. Indeed, if medicine is not for you, you may not even recognise that fantastic experiences even occur. For those entering medical school straight after leaving secondary school, the process of growing up, leaving home and living in a different environment changes their priorities so greatly that medical school no longer has a place in their lives.

Students who do decide medicine is no longer the correct career choice for them can expect to be supported by their medical school in obtaining an alternative degree at the end of three years or in transferring to another course.[3] Seek advice from careers advisors and tutors about your options.

SUPPORT FOR MEDICAL STUDENTS

> Students must have appropriate support for their academic and general welfare needs at all stages.[3]

Medical students should be supported through stress or emotional, financial or academic troubles and in seeking appropriate help.[4] Medical schools have a duty to produce clear information about the support available, including that at clinical placements at sites other than your base hospital (the hospital directly linked to your medical school). You are entitled to privacy, equal opportunity and adequate support and representation on a daily basis and at times of need. Standards have been set out by the Council of Heads of Medical Schools (CHMS) and the British Medical Association Medical Students Committee (BMA MSC) to ensure that your medical school provides you with adequate privacy, equal opportunity, support and representation. These standards have been summarised in Appendix V.

Most medical students believe their welfare needs are adequately met by their medical school/faculty at their higher education institution.[5] This is good news; however, in order to seek help you need to be aware of what is available, when and from where. Universities support their students well, offering support, service and/

or advice centres which contain disability, finance, counselling, accommodation, employment and international offices. Thus many of the issues you may face while studying are managed at such centres.

Educational

Your educational progress should be supported from the beginning; specifically, before you get into difficulties. Medical schools should provide you with guidance about your core curriculum, student-selected components and assessments.[3] Course handbooks will usually contain this information. Knowing what is expected of you will prevent difficulties before they arise and understanding applicable policies and procedures will help if you do start to struggle.

Undergraduate medical degrees are designed to be challenging. Integrated time for reflection and personal growth (e.g. study periods and 'holidays') can be used to catch up if you have missed any work due to illness or other good personal reasons. Even if you have not been absent, this personal time can be used to reach a higher level of understanding.

If you are having difficulty in one particular subject, you should have access to a named person to deal with this. Talk to your tutors to find out how to contact the appropriate person.

Medical schools will help you to monitor and assess your progress by providing you with logbooks, portfolios and/or self-assessments. Assessment forms that are completed by healthcare staff on clinical attachments will provide guidance on your progress. However, only you know what you find difficult, if you are struggling or if you need extra help. The responsibility to frequently reflect on your educational progress and seek help if needed falls on your shoulders.

Medical schools will provide you with support and feedback if you struggle academically. This support should occur within two weeks of the problem being identified.[6] The earlier you seek help, the earlier it will be sorted, and the higher the chance is of a resolution.

Financial

Medical schools must provide information on internal and external sources of funding.[6] Often, student support centres and/or student unions contain financial advice offices or departments. They will know about specific scholarships and bursaries available to you, as well as more nationwide schemes and providers. You will find more information on sources of financial help and how to handle your money in Chapter 11.

Emotional
Friends and family

Your friends and family are invaluable during medical school. Keep in touch with them regularly, be there for them and they will be there for you. Your old friends will soon lose interest if you only phone them to have a moan. Life will always seem easier if you have the support of friends and family.

Tutors and wardens

Tutors are a common source of support to medical students. Up to 75% of medical students have a tutor within their medical school with whom they feel they can share welfare concerns.[5] Tutors are usually academic members of staff so can usually help you with academic and non-academic issues. The most important qualities of tutors are that they are:[4]

➡ available, approachable and enthusiastic
➡ compassionate, empathetic, encouraging
➡ knowledgeable, experienced
➡ fair
➡ independent from academic issues
➡ respect confidentiality
➡ have enough time to provide adequate support.

Wardens are not always available and are usually associated with campus accommodation. However, their role, when present, can include support for non-academic and welfare issues. Find out about the availability of wardens before you have any issues to make it easier to seek help in times of distress.

University counselling services

University student support centres and/or student unions usually contain a university-based counselling service which provides confidential, free counselling. Other university-based counselling services can include Nightline, usually advertised around the university (especially in toilets). Nightline is a free/cheap-rate phone line that you can ring if you are having emotional difficulties during evening/night time hours. Some Nightline services have email and telephone lines.

Mentors

> The process whereby an experienced, highly regarded, empathic person (the mentor) guides another individual (the mentee) in the development and re-examination of their own ideas, learning, and personal and professional development. The mentor, who often, but not necessarily, works in the same organisation or field as the mentee, achieves this by listening and talking in confidence to the mentee.[7]

The BMA advocates mentoring at every level of medical education and careers.[8] Mentors take many forms. Your medical school may have interpersonal or e-mentoring schemes; the latter being conducted over the internet. Your mentor may be in the year above (sometimes known as 'mummy' or 'daddy'), or a more experienced individual who knows what you are going through and has come out the other end.

Choose your mentor well. They must be someone you trust and with whom you feel comfortable and communicate well.

Health and well-being

> Medical students . . . are susceptible to a particular range of health problems, including depression and substance misuse . . . the selection process for medical schools may favour individuals with perfectionist, obsessive-compulsive, self-critical and altruistic traits, all of which predispose to vulnerability to psychological illness.[9]

Just as doctors are expected to maintain their health to the optimum level, medical students must do the same. Maintenance of your health includes eating and sleeping adequately, seeking medical attention when ill and maintaining contemporary records with occupational health departments. Box 14.1 illustrates how your well-being, or lack of it, can affect your fitness to practice as a doctor.

> **Box 14.1 Factors that may result in a medical student being deemed unfit for practice[10]**
> - Severe physical or mental health problems can put patient safety in jeopardy, including infectious diseases
> - Personal misconduct, including dishonesty and plagiarism
> - Substance misuse
> - Criminal conviction

Trusts produce local policies to protect you and your patients' safety. Medical students should pay particular attention to policies covering moving and handling of patients, sharps disposal, infection control, personal protective equipment and fire and security procedures. For further details speak to your tutors or occupational health department and/or look on the hospital intranet.

Medical schools stress the importance of registration with a GP and should inform you of occupational health and counselling services.[3] If your health (mental or physical) deteriorates, or if you become involved with drug or alcohol misuse, you have the same right to confidentiality as any other patient (i.e. confidentiality must be maintained unless there is risk of death or serious harm to others).[3] Some universities automatically register students with local GP practices, but this is an exception, not the rule. Investigate and register at local GP practices during the early days at university.

When you go to university, take with you your medical card (unless you are an overseas student) and vaccination records. If you take regular medications, bring enough with you to last you two to four months to allow adequate time to find a GP and register. These simple steps will make registration and information transfer to your new GP easier.

University-based health centres

Universities have their own health centres with which you can register if you are a student and/or living in the local area. Health centres usually house GPs, nurses and counsellors and thus are adequate for minor health needs (i.e. not requiring hospital treatment) during term time. However university-based health centres are usually shut during holidays. If you live in the area of your university, register at a local GP or non-university-based health centre that you can access during holiday periods. Other services sometimes offered by university health centres include travel and contraception advice and complementary therapy.

Occupational health departments

While at university you will usually be under the care of the university occupational health department; once you qualify your care transfers to the hospital/trust occupational health department. Each time you register at a new occupational health department you need to present information on your immunisation history and immunity status. Unless your hospital and/or medical school uses NHS personal data cards, cards containing your contact details, professional registration status and occupational health and immunisation records, you will be required to provide evidence of the immunisations you have received and evidence of your hepatitis B/C status (i.e. do you have hepatitis B/C). Keep all relevant laboratory blood (or other relevant) reports safe. If you can, scan your laboratory results onto your computer so you can easily print out copies when required.

Stress

> Medical students report higher levels of psychological symptoms than the general population. Levels of distress increase progressively during the course. Students perceived the need for personal healthcare, but 'feared reprisal for seeking help'.[11]

Stress is complex and an increasingly common problem.[12] Stress has a moderate effect on up to 50% of medical students. and an extreme impact on the health of one in ten medical students. Medical students' stress is attributable to a number of causes, for example:[4]

➡ heavy workload

➡ financial concerns; having to do paid work to make ends meet

➡ family and/or domestic responsibilities
➡ change of culture
➡ exams
➡ fear of failing or not doing well
➡ differences in personality types or coping mechanisms[13]
➡ variability in the provision or use of support systems[13]
➡ competitiveness versus co-operation[14]
➡ living in an unfamiliar environment a long way from normal social supports and/or familiar culture.

How do you know if you are suffering from the effects of stress? The symptoms of stress vary widely; Minck describes them as follows.[12] Mild stress may result in insomnia, sweating, palpitations, muscle tension, appetite change and digestive disturbances. As stress becomes worse you can suffer from hypersensitivity to sensory stimuli, personality change in others' eyes, distractibility, increased use of alcohol or tobacco and even thoughts of quitting medical school or personal relationships.[12]

Learn to manage stress in a healthy and constructive way. Throughout your career you will be expected to work hard and well through times of great stress. If you learn ineffective coping mechanisms now, you will find it difficult to change later on. If you are stressed because you are working too hard, try and cut down on what you are doing or at least the amount of time you spend working. Reduce the expectations you have for yourself and realise that you cannot do everything.[12]

Do not suffer in silence

Medical schools must give consideration to extenuating circumstances that (potentially) affect your progress. If illness, family pressures or other circumstances result in serious problems you should inform your medical school, perhaps via a trusted tutor.

> I became ill in my second year. I was hospitalised for two weeks just before an assessed presentation and was ill for a number of months over an exam period. I told my medical school as soon as I knew the problem wasn't going to be sorted quickly. They told me that if I took my upcoming exams and failed they wouldn't count them as a first attempt. It allowed me to attempt the exams, but took the pressure off me in the event that I failed. (*Lizzie Cottrell, fifth-year medical student, Manchester*)

Some doctors and medical students find it difficult to seek help when they become mentally or physically ill, thus ensues a feeling of isolation and reluctance to take time off when needed. Primary prevention is key; prevent your mental and physical health deteriorating while in medical school and beyond by following some basic tips.

� Seek help when required and seek it early.

➾ Eat a healthy balanced diet and drink plenty of non-alcoholic, caffeine-free drinks.

➾ Sleep adequately. Insufficient sleep will affect you in the short term by reducing your energy levels and concentration and in the long term, e.g. predisposing you to high blood pressure.[14]

➾ Exercise to reduce stress and increase positive feelings.

➾ Maintain useful, mutually supportive friendships.

➾ Be open with yourself and others about feelings, problems, stresses and happiness.

➾ Spend adequate time doing something you enjoy. Make sure that work and other responsibilities do not take over.

Medical students and eating disorders

> **People with disordered eating are often sensitive, perfectionists and high achievers. Is it any wonder, then, that medical schools seem to be full of them?[15]**

Nearly 20% of female medical students suffer from disordered eating.[16] Worryingly, medical students with disordered eating typically present late, as they fear negative effects on their career. However, well-timed presentation can result in effective treatment and good recovery. If you are worried that you or a friend are suffering from an eating disorder help and advice is available.

Disordered eating encompasses two main disorders; anorexia nervosa and bulimia nervosa. Individuals with anorexia nervosa believe that they are overweight. In an attempt to overcome this they take drastic measures to reduce their weight by reducing food intake and/or using compensatory methods to get rid of food/water (e.g. abuse of laxatives/diuretics) or fat (e.g. excessive exercise). Such individuals fail to maintain a 'normal' body weight and thus experience physical effects such as cessation of menstruation.

Bulimia nervosa is a disorder in which weight loss is not a predominant feature. People with bulimia characteristically binge on large quantities of food and compensate for this by inducing vomiting, taking laxatives, reducing food and/or exercising excessively.

Eating disorders are a manifestation of low self-esteem and illustrate a desire for control over life or emotion. Medical students are usually hard-driven individuals who are commonly perfectionists. These traits increase the risk of eating disorders. Controlling food intake and/or losing weight may reward the individual's success in this self-set task.

Restricted or fluctuating food intake reduces the ability to think and study effectively. Affective (e.g. depression and anxiety) disorders occur in most people with anorexia nervosa during their lifetime; a third of people with anorexia nervosa suffer with severe depression.[16] Some eating disorders are associated with an increased risk of drug and alcohol abuse.

The physical effects of disordered eating can lead to an increased risk of injury, salt disturbances in the body and heart failure in some cases.[16] These extreme negative effects on (mental and physical) health demonstrate the importance of you being vigilant for signs of eating disorders in yourself and your colleagues. Importantly, you have a responsibility to yourself and your patients.

Eating disorders do not always produce super-thin, skeletal-like people. Even if weight loss is a feature, this is often concealed with baggy or layered clothing. What are the signs of disordered eating? Medical students spend lots of time working together. Clues may be demonstrated from your colleagues' behaviour to indicate they have disordered eating; for example:

➡ missing lunch using excuses of work, study or clinical experience
➡ quickly leaving to go to the toilet after eating
➡ not wanting to attend food-centred socials
➡ fainting at unusual times, such as on a ward round when it is not hot/ gruesome.

If you want information, advice or support for yourself or a friend with an eating disorder, help is out there. Make sure you seek it promptly.

Drug- and alcohol-related problems

Drug- and alcohol-related problems are important for medical students. At least 20% of medical students use alcohol to cope with the pressures of medical school,[5] 50% of medical students exceed the World Health Organization guidelines for safe limits of alcohol consumption[11] and three-quarters believe that drugs or alcohol negatively affects the medical school culture.[5] The use of drugs and alcohol by medical students or healthcare professionals puts the health of patients at risk. Thus, drug- and alcohol-related problems must be taken very seriously.

Medical schools can refuse to graduate students who misuse drugs or alcohol. However, they are required to support and counsel such students with the aim of helping them to graduate in the future.[4] For those of you who have (or know someone who has) a problem with alcohol/drug dependency, (encourage them to) seek help immediately. The good news is that doctors and nurses tend to do well in treatment.[17] Effective help, once the need is identified, is out there.

External sources of help

You may have unsuccessfully tried your university, medical school, tutors, friends and/or family for support, or felt this is inappropriate. If this is the case, a number of external sources of help may be useful. A brief overview of the variety of support on offer to you as a medical student and as a doctor ensues.

British Medical Association

The British Medical Association (BMA) runs a counselling service for its members (including students) and their families. The counselling service is a 24-hour support service that eligible individuals may access an unlimited number of times. Counsellors, who work strictly within the bounds of confidentiality, are trained to provide assistance for emotional, personal and work-related problems.

Support4doctors

Support4doctors (www.support4doctors), set up by the Royal Medical Benevolent Fund, is a useful starting point if things go wrong when you are a medical student/ doctor. A quick web guide provides links to nearly a hundred different helpful organisations and resources. All you have to do is log on. Membership or passwords are not required. The site is organised under four main headings – work and career, money and finance, family and home, and health and well-being.

Doctors' Support Network

The Doctors' Support Network (DSN) is a warm, friendly self-help group for doctors and medical students with mental health concerns, including stress, burn-out, anxiety, depression, manic depression, psychoses and eating disorders. The group believes that contact with (and support from) other doctors can aid recovery. All doctors in the group have been troubled at some stage in their lives. Thus the group is well placed to help those who are beginning the slow process of re-establishing themselves after a breakdown or other mental crisis. The DSN also believes that appropriate support offered before a crisis develops helps to defuse it. The DSN seeks to reduce the isolation and stigma associated with mental health concerns. It is not group therapy, nor does it have other therapeutic aims. It aims to complement other sources of support available to doctors and fills a gap not otherwise catered for. The DSN has regular meetings throughout the UK. Members also receive a regular newsletter and have access to a lively email discussion group. Medical students have their own group (and membership) within DSN.

Doctor's SupportLine

Losing your balance? Exam stress? Depression? Worries at home? Anxiety? Wondering if you are going to make it? The Doctor's SupportLine is a helpline that offers you a chance to talk things through informally and in complete confidence with someone who has been there and got the t-shirt; a trained, volunteer doctor. Both volunteers and callers remain anonymous, so you can be reassured nothing will be passed on. This is an independent organisation with charitable status, offering friendly, non-judgemental support to UK doctors and medical students.

If you want to seek emotional support from a non-medicine-related organisation, the Samaritans may be a good choice. Samaritans services are available 24 hours a day and are provided by nearly 16 000 trained volunteers. Samaritans provide confidential emotional support for anybody experiencing feelings of distress or despair, including those that may lead to suicide. Samaritans offer a support helpline for people in distress. The charity should not be viewed as the last stop but as a first port of call. It is important to realise Samaritans are not just about suicide. Although Samaritans does aim to reduce the number of deaths by suicide, they also recognise that good emotional health is the key to a successful society. For you, good emotional health will also be the key to a successful time at medical school and a promising medical career.

FITNESS TO PRACTICE[10]

Medical schools have to assess medical students' fitness to practice. The GMC's increasing involvement in this may result in those who are unfit to practice losing their place at medical school. Factors that affect fitness to practice were shown earlier in Box 14.1.

Should your fitness to practice be questioned, you may face suspension from your studies and you will be brought in front of a fitness to practice committee to discuss the issue(s) of concern. Such a panel consists of senior medical school staff (e.g. the dean), healthcare professionals (GPs, consultants, junior doctors), an observer (university professional from a different faculty), medical student and a non-medical chair. Your defence union and the BMA (if you are a member) can be important sources of advice and support at this time.

Fitness to practice committee hearings usually result in one of three outcomes:
➡ no further action
➡ continuation of study but extra action is required; resubmission of work, regular health reviews, re-sitting exams
➡ you are withdrawn from your medical course; in this case you may be directed to an alternative course.

FURTHER SCENARIOS

You will find advice on the following situations in *The Medical Student's Survival Guide 2: going clinical*:
➡ what to do if you have a problem with your medical team
➡ restriction of religious practices
➡ assessing and managing deteriorating patients and emergencies
➡ coping with patients dying
➡ mistakes
➡ needlestick injury.

FURTHER READING

Anonymous. Living with Ed. *StudentBMJ*. 2005; **13**: 163. (A medical student's account of living with an eating disorder, Part 1.)

Anonymous. Surviving Ed. *StudentBMJ*. 2006; **14**: 167. (A medical student's account of living with an eating disorder, Part 2.)

Anorexia and Bulimia Care. (www.anorexiabulimiacare.co.uk)

British Medical Association. *BMA Doctors for Doctors*. (Available at: www.bma.org.uk) (A web-based self-help tool aimed to assist doctors in accessing appropriate help for difficulties they may be facing.)

Eating Disorders Association. (www.edauk.com)

Harwood I, Stansfeld S. Doctors and alcohol misuse. *StudentBMJ*. 2006; **14**: 276.

Houghton A. Personal support 5: stress and time management for people with multiple responsibilities. *BMJ Career Focus*. 2005; **331**: 30.

Janes C. People power. *BMJ Careers*. 2006; **333**: 143–4.

www.mentalhealth.org.uk (Contains information on and sources of support for various mental health problems from alcohol addiction problems to Alzheimer's disease. If you want a source of reference, or to find appropriate help, this website may be a good starting point.)

Sick Doctors Trust (www.sick-doctors-trust.co.uk)

Somerset & Wessex Eating Disorders Association: 18–25 Project. (www.sweda18-25.org.uk) (Includes a section on going to university with an eating disorder.)

Tynan A. *Pushing the Boat Out: an introductory study of admissions to UK medical, dental and veterinary schools for applicants with disabilities*. 2003. (Available at: www.ltsn-01.ac.uk/ltsn_images/pdfs/ptbo_final.pdf)

Yadthore S. Tips on . . . coping with exam failure. *BMJ Careers*. 2006; **333**: 156.

CHAPTER 15

How to get the most from medical school

Over 60 specialties exist in medicine and surgery, each with their own sub-specialties. It is impossible for medical school curricula to incorporate all specialties. Therefore, self-selected components of the course and self-directed extra-curricular activity enable further (or new) experience of the specialties that interest you or are an area of personal weakness. So how do you make your medical training as useful, broad and full of variety as possible?

Optional components of the medical degree may be formally arranged into projects or the elective period (*see The Medical Student's Survival Guide 2: going clinical*). However, you may wish to undertake additional experience independently. Use your initiative to pursue your interests while you still have the freedom of being a medical student.

STUDENT-SELECTED COMPONENTS

> The core curriculum must be supported by a series of student-selected components that allow students to study, in depth, any areas of particular interest to them.[1]

Student-selected components (SSCs) are a requirement of an undergraduate medical degree. SSCs enable you to study areas of medicine in greater depth than your medical degree would normally allow. SSCs should comprise a quarter to one-third of your degree period.[1] SSCs do not all have to be clinical; however, all must be medical-related – this encompasses laboratory-based, biological, research-oriented, history of medicine, behavioural and psychosocial-related areas.

In some medical schools the term 'student-selected component' may be replaced with:

➡ special study module (SSM)
➡ selected study component (SSC)
➡ special study unit (SSU).

SSCs are undertaken over a couple to a few weeks. During this time you will focus on a specific topic and produce a final report. You are expected to study literature and gain experience in the area you have chosen.

A personal tutor will oversee your project. Meet with your tutor prior to starting your project to discuss what the project will involve and any appropriate preparatory work. Arrange regular meetings with your tutor throughout the project period to enable you to ask plenty of questions and to allow your tutor to gauge your enthusiasm and/or stage of learning in order to stretch you or make you aware of further experiences as appropriate.

Aims of an SSC

So what should you be trying to achieve while undertaking SSCs? You, your medical school and/or your tutor set objectives to encourage you to get the richest experience possible. Aims of medical school SSCs are for you to:[1]

➡ study a topic in greater depth than you can during your core-curriculum activities
➡ become proficient at presenting work in written format and via oral presentations
➡ develop skills that help you to critically analyse healthcare systems, treatments and care of patients
➡ learn, develop and master research and evidence-based medicine skills
➡ learn, practise, develop and use skills
➡ consider new career paths, or evaluate pre-existing career choices.

Choosing an SSC

SSCs provide fantastic opportunities for you to be able to access experiences that become more unobtainable post-graduation. The broader experience they provide will give you a better foundation on which to build your future career decisions.

When choosing an SSC, think about the following.

➡ What interests you?
➡ What are your weak areas?
➡ Which topics are neglected by the core curriculum?

You will undertake a number of SSCs during medical school; pick a variety of topics and specialties. If you are interested in a specific career, use SSCs to experience a variety of specialties that will provide useful and relevant skills and experience. You may be introduced to an area of medicine that you enjoy but have never before considered.

You may have to devise your own project or choose from a list. Medical schools often hold information on available and/or previous SSC projects. Have a look at what previous students have done to give you ideas. If there is something you really want to do and it is not on the list, make enquiries about designing your own SSC with the medical school and identify a potential tutor.

If you set your own project, make sure it is not too broad. By all means experience a broad range of skills and situations during your SSC, but your project will only be allowed a limited number of words. You want to be able to demonstrate your writing, research, analytical and appraisal skills within your project. If your topic is too broad you will not be able to involve these skills to any great extent and you may not be able to demonstrate your true colours accurately.

SSC assessment

Your performance, diligence, enthusiasm and understanding during your SSC will be assessed. Your written report will demonstrate your evidence-based medicine and writing skills. Oral presentations of your project and/or findings may be assessed for the clarity of your communication and your ability to summarise your project concisely.

Your medical school may provide the following assessment forms:
➡ activity diary: provides evidence of what you spent your time doing
➡ attendance report
➡ performance and attitude report.

Some students look at SSCs as a bit of a holiday but this is a waste of a valuable time. Make the most of the opportunity you have been provided with to really get involved in an area of medicine you may otherwise have graduated knowing little about.

ETHICS

Ethics should always be at the forefront of all healthcare professionals' minds. It is important that all individuals involved in providing patient care behave ethically. Ethical practice improves doctor–patient relationships and public perception of healthcare.

Although ethical topics are deeply and broadly included in your core curriculum, expand on these independently. Reflect on your experiences, each day or week. Think of an ethical dilemma that has arisen and consult relevant publications from the GMC (www.gmc-uk.org) and the BMA (www.bma.org.uk) for official guidance. Determine the extent to which the guidance was followed. Were there any deviations? Why? How would you handle the same situation in the future? This process will refine your reflection skills and help you to learn ethical principles in a memorable way.

Ethical debates or lectures are often organised in addition to the medical student curriculum. Some hospitals/departments hold lunchtime/evening meetings at which a hot topic is discussed. An external lecturer or speaker may be invited to hold a discussion or lecture. Attend these events whenever possible. You may gain a new perspective from considering the views of practising doctors and other healthcare professionals.

CHAPTER 16

Looking forward

You are at medical school to learn the basics of undertaking a career in medicine. Throughout medical school you should develop the skills a doctor needs to practise clinical medicine and those that are required to be successful in getting a job. Think about your career early: you do not need to plan your specialty, but think about a rough area that interests you and how you can impress an application panel to give you the passport into any career you desire.

PREPARATION FOR JOB APPLICATIONS: YOUR CAREER COUNTDOWN

> **You are unique and so is everyone else.**

Early preparation is the key to a successful career. When you first enter medical school it is easy to become complacent about your career. However, there is tough competition ahead. Make yourself stand out from everyone else (who are all trying to do the same). Below is a guide to help you prepare for future job applications and a successful career from your first year at medical school.

Pre-clinical years

Use your pre-clinical/early years to build good foundations for your future knowledge. If you do not learn the basics at this stage you will have difficulty in understanding even basic clinical information. It is easy to fall into a lazy student life.

In addition to working hard, play hard and learn to take 'time out'. Learn healthy study habits, including taking rests, breaks and days off. Develop interests away from medicine. Joining a club or society will give you prescribed time away from your study. Interests away from medicine will provide a good distraction when things get tough in the future and will also give you something to put on your future job applications.

'Fun' activities and interests may be deciding factors in future job applications. The pressure is on to have the most interesting and diverse hobbies; but this may be unfounded. Rather than thinking about which hobbies will make you stand out, think about the hobbies and non-medical activities you enjoy, and identify how they may inform or assist your future medical career. Make these links early and filling in your job applications will be easier as your answers will be clear, thoughtful and true.

Grab every opportunity. Get involved in projects or committees. Attending extra-curricular lectures will demonstrate your enthusiasm. They may also result in publications or improved exam results. Whatever it is, if you are interested, give it a go. Be open to experiences at this early stage; the workshop you recently attended may have been the introduction to your future career

Take advantage of your long summer (Christmas and Easter!) holidays by resting but also undertaking part-time work. Progression through medical school lengthens your academic years and increases demands from your work and your levels of tiredness. Part-time jobs could be medical-related (*see* Chapter 11). Whatever you do, work will give you a bit of extra cash to last you through the forthcoming year.

Take student-selected components (SSCs, *see* Chapter 15) seriously. Choose varied topics that interest you and work hard. SSCs are designed, in your pre-clinical years, to give you the skills required to undertake evidence-based medicine and to succeed at writing reports and publications in the future. They are also an opportunity to get a taste of the specialty that interests you for your future career at this stage. It may provide valuable information on whether or not it is actually the career for you. A final reason to take SSCs seriously is that the grades you obtain for your projects may count towards your grading from your medical school when you are applying for your junior doctor job.

Compile a record of professional development (ROPD). If you have not started one yet, do so immediately. It must be up-to-date at every point of your medical school career. You may be given a folder in which to place such information; if not, designate a large, lever arch file into which you can put your professional development information. Collate exam results, extra copies of your written reports, grades / marks for assessments and include a copy of your CV. As you progress through medical school and accumulate information, grades, certificates and publications, all you have to do is add these to the file as they occur. Even if you do not use a CV to apply for your first postgraduate jobs, having information organised in this way will help you complete application forms.

What do you want to do in your future career? Do you want to be a GP, hospital physician, surgeon or laboratory-based? These are broad but narrow enough choices for the time being. Have you ever thought about yourself? What do you enjoy doing? What work–life balance do you desire? As you progress through medical school, use clinical experiences and personal reflection to narrow your favourite category to favourite and appropriate sub-specialties. If you know what you want to be at this stage, try and remain open-minded and experience other specialties. You may discover something else you like and had previously not considered; or it may confirm your intentions are right for you. Wide experience at this early stage is always useful, as patients never have problems just relating to one specialty, for example vascular surgeons have to manage patients having asthma attacks while under their care.

Epilogue

If you have bought this book you have shown you want to help yourself to go far. This demonstrates the right mindset for any future or current doctor. Keep this up – no one else is responsible for your career apart from you.

Gain further information on surviving the rest of your course and career from *The Medical Student's Survival Guide 2: going clinical*. This book contains information on:

➡ the clinical years
➡ talking with patients and colleagues
➡ history-taking, examination and presentation of patients
➡ ward life and rounds
➡ clinic, theatre and community placements
➡ how to get the most from the clinical years
➡ electives
➡ when things go wrong in the clinical setting
➡ difficult individuals and life after medical school.

Finally, I want to wish you luck. The hard work is worth it in the end. With the right attitude, adequate knowledge and regular reflection you will go far and, I hope, enjoy being a doctor as much as I do.

Resources

MEDICAL SCHOOL: THE EARLY DAYS

Medical Protection Society
Granary Wharf House
Leeds LS11 5PY
Tel: 9845 900 0022
Website: www.mps.org.uk/student

Medical and Dental Defence Union of Scotland
Mackintosh House
120 Blythswood Street
Glasgow G2 4EA
Tel: 0141 221 5858
Website: www.mddus.com

LEARNING

BMJ Learning
E-mail: bmjlearning@bmjgroup.com
Website: www.bmjlearning.com

Professional Medical Education
Tel: 0800 043 2060
E-mail: courses@freefees.co.uk
Website: www.freefees.co.uk

EXAMS

Professional Medical Education
Tel: 0800 043 2060
E-mail: courses@freefees.co.uk
Website: www.freefees.co.uk

LET'S TALK MONEY

BMA Medical Education Trust
BMA Charities
BMA House
Tavistock Square
London WC1H 9JP
E-mail: info.bmacharities@bma.org.uk

Department of Employment, Learning, Training
Student Support Branch
4th Floor
Adelaide House
39–49 Adelaide Street
Belfast BT2 8FD
Tel: 0289 025 7777

Professional Medical Education/Finance
Tel: 0800 043 2060
E-mail: info@freefees.co.uk
Website: www.freefees.co.uk

NHS Student Grants Unit
Hesketh House
200–220 Broadway
Fleetwood FY7 8SS
Tel: 0845 358 6655
Website: www.nhsstudentgrants.co.uk

NHS (Wales) Student Awards Unit
2nd Floor
Golate House
101 St Mary Street
Cardiff CF10 1DX
Tel: 0292 026 1495

Student Awards Agency for Scotland
Gyle View House
3 Redheughs Rigg
South Gyle
Edinburgh EH12 9HH
Tel: 0131 476 8212
Website: www.saas.gov.uk

Student Loans Company Ltd
100 Bothwell Street
Glasgow G2 7JD
Tel: 0800 405010
Website: www.slc.co.uk

Wesleyan Medical Sickness
Colmore Circus
Birmingham B4 6AR
Tel: 0800 358 6060
Website: www.wesleyanmedicalsickness.co.uk

LIFE AWAY FROM MEDICINE

www.clubeasy.com
www.easyroommate.com
www.fish4lettings.com
www.flatmateclick.co.uk
www.spareroom.co.uk

Medics on the move
Bridge House
8 Avon Vale
Stoke Bishop
Bristol BS9 1TB
Tel: 0870 350 1858
E-mail: info@medicsonthemove.co.uk
Website: www.medicsonthemove.co.uk

WHEN THINGS GO WRONG

Anorexia Bulimia Care (ABC)
PO Box 173
Letchworth
Herts SG6 1XQ
Tel: 0146 242 3351
E-mail: anorexiabulimiacare@ntlworld.com
Website: www.anorexiabulimiacare.co.uk

BMA Counselling Service
Tel: 0845 920 0169 (Local rates apply; open anytime, day or night, 365 days a year)

BMA Doctors for Doctors Unit
Tel: 020 7383 6739

Doctors' SupportLine
38 Harwood Road
London SW6 4PH
Tel: 0870 765 0001 (Generally open at the following times: Mon–Tue 6 pm to 11 pm;
Wed–Fri 6 pm to 10 pm; Sun 10 am to 10 pm; Sat closed)
Website: www.doctorssupport.org

Doctors' Support Network (DSN)
PO Box 360
Stevenage SG1 9AS
Tel: 0870 321 0642
Website: www.dsn.org.uk

Doctors' Support Network (DSN) Wales and South-west
5 Borage Close
Pontprennaeu
Cardiff CF23 8SJ
Tel: 0870 321 0642 or 0292 073 1025 (for administrative enquiries)

Eating Disorders Association
103 Prince of Wales Road
Norwich NR1 1DW
Tel: 0845 634 1414 (helpline) or 0870 770 3256 (for administrative enquiries)
E-mail: infor@edauk.com
Website: www.edauk.com

Mental Health Foundation
Website: www.mentalhealth.org.uk

Mind – mental health charity in England and Wales
Tel: 0845 766 0163
Website: www.mind.org.uk

Samaritans
PO Box 9090
Stirling FK8 2SA
Tel: 0845 790 9090; 185 060 9090 (Republic of Ireland)
Website: www.samaritans.org.uk

Sick Doctors Trust
Tel: 0870 444 5163
Website: www.sick-doctors-trust.co.uk

Support4Doctors
Website: www.support4doctors.org

APPENDIX II

Standards relating to attitude and behaviour

Council of Heads of Medical Schools and British Medical Association Medical Students Committee. *Medical Student Charter, 2005*. (Available at: www.bma.org. uk/ap.nsf/Content/MedSchCharter)

Standard	Details and further expectations
The student will treat every patient politely and considerately	Treat every patient with respect. Be prepared to respond to a patient's individual needs. Ensure the patient understands you are a student and not a qualified doctor. Take steps to overcome any barriers to communication. Make sure the patient agrees to your presence and involvement. Set aside personal and cultural preferences. Do not continue if the patient indicates a wish for you to stop. Maintain an appropriate general appearance, facial expression and other non-verbal signs. Dress appropriately – not too informal or at the extremes of fashion. Acknowledge that you are expected to appear and be professional.
The student will respect patients' dignity and privacy	Address patients in a professional way. Address patients formally until given specific permission by the patient to be more informal. Endeavour to preserve the patient's dignity at all times. Attempt to ensure the patient's privacy at all times.
The student will listen to patients and respect their views	Do not ignore what the patient has to say. Do not interrogate the patient when taking a history.
The student will take of the opportunities provided to develop his/her professional knowledge and skills	Attend all compulsory teaching sessions, or, if unable to attend, inform the medical school as soon as possible of the reason for absence. Keep professional knowledge and skills up to date. Complete and submit work on time. Read up on patients you have seen. Be conscientious. Practise your clinical skills. Endeavour to contribute effectively to learning groups. Respond positively to reasonable feedback.
The student will take of the opportunities provided to develop his/her professional knowledge and skills (cont.)	Immediately inform medical school of factors that may affect your performance to allow appropriate action to be taken. Carry out examinations (including intimate examinations where necessary and with a chaperone) on patients of both sexes.

(continued)

Standard	Details and further expectations
The student will recognise the limits of his/her professional competence	Do not hesitate to ask for help and advice when necessary. Do not undertake tasks or give advice beyond your level of competence.
The student will be honest and trustworthy in all matters	All forms of academic cheating and plagiarism are unacceptable and may result in disciplinary proceedings. If you are not trustworthy in your academic life it will be difficult to be trustworthy in a clinical setting. You should be given a copy of information about the disciplinary proceedings for your medical school.
The student will respect and protect confidential information	Do not deliberately divulge information concerning a patient to anyone not directly involved in their care. You will have access to information that the patients will expect to be kept confidential. Do not discuss patients in a public place and take other precautions to ensure inadvertent passing of information about a patient does not occur.
Students must not allow their personal beliefs to prejudice their patients' care	Care for patients irrespective of your views on their lifestyles, culture, religion, beliefs, race, colour, gender, sexuality, disability, age, nationality or social or economic status.
Students will act quickly to protect patients from risk if they have good reason to believe that they or a colleague may not be fit to practice	The student will immediately report any concerns to a senior member of staff using the procedures for complaints and whistle-blowing assigned by the medical school. If necessary contact a professional organisation or the GMC for advice.
The student will work with colleagues in the ways that best serve the patients' interests	Acknowledge that healthcare is dependent on effective co-operation between all team members. Attempt to ensure you maintain good relationships with other health professionals caring for the patients. Treat other healthcare professionals, staff, other members of the university and fellow students with respect.
The student undertakes to provide feedback on the usefulness, significance and effectiveness of all aspects of the course, including teaching	–

Standards medical schools are expected to meet regarding education, training and facilities

Council of Heads of Medical Schools and British Medical Association Medical Students Committee. *Medical Student Charter, 2005*. (Available at: www.bma.org. uk/ap.nsf/Content/MedSchCharter)

Standard: your medical school should . . .	Further details of the standards that should be met by the medical school
Provide high-quality teaching and training in clinical and non-clinical settings	Your medical school is obliged to comply with the General Medical Council (GMC) document, *Tomorrow's Doctors*[1]
	This standard is assessed by the GMC quality assurance visiting process, but should also be a proactive duty of the medical school
	Students should be involved, where possible, in the quality assurance process
Provide clear learning objectives and outcomes, around which teaching is structured	The learning objectives and outcomes should be clear and easily accessible to you
Ensure assessment and examinations are based upon the learning objectives and outcomes	This standard aims to ensure continuity and fairness
	Your assessments and examinations will be based upon the GMC standards and your medical school syllabus
Provide learning experiences that are challenging and stimulating	–
Ensure that staff and students understand their responsibilities with respect to gaining consent from patients prior to examinations by students	–

(continued)

Standard: your medical school should . . .	Further details of the standards that should be met by the medical school
Provide a level of training whereby, upon completion of the course, the minimum standards attained comply with the professional expectations of the regulating body	All courses, and changes to courses, must be approved by the GMC
Make clear the responsibilities and expectations of the regulating body and how they relate to the curriculum; the professional duties of the regulating body must be made known to the students	Fitness to practice and professional duties are important features of the curriculum; the medical schools should make these, and the implications of these, clear to you
Ensure that the course is relevant and led by individuals qualified to teach and train undergraduate medical students	
Give impartial, timely and constructive feedback on individual student progress and performance, including explanations for failure	Expect to be told and be given constructive feedback and support if you are failing to meet academic standards at any stage of your course (within two weeks of the problem being identified)
Provide access to extra support and advice from teachers and tutors	
Inform, regularly update and provide access to full information about the course, module contents and course objectives	Your medical school should clearly communicate changes to and information regarding your course Communication and dissemination of information may be facilitated by student representatives
Give clear and timely information about assessment/submission dates and the preferred or required format of assessments or submissions	Clear assessment dates and formats Expect at least one month's prior warning of assessments
Provide timetabled information about the academic year at least one month before commencement of the year	–
Details about external placements should be provided at least one month before commencement of the placement	–
Ensure that students have easy access to sample/past examination papers and other relevant examination resources	–

(continued)

Standard: your medical school should . . .	Further details of the standards that should be met by the medical school
Where requested, give due consideration to extenuating circumstances which may affect academic and clinical progress and performance in any aspect of the medical course	Extenuating circumstances may include family pressures, illness and personal circumstances Your medical school must be aware of its requirements under the Disability Discrimination Act (www.opsi.gov.uk/acts/acts1995/1995050.htm) and make reasonable adjustments where necessary
Wherever possible, provide students with the opportunity to study and practice abroad as part of the medical degree	International schemes such as ERASMUS (www.erasmus.ac.uk) offer the opportunity to study modules or for student-selected components (SSCs) abroad
Respect the intellectual property rights of the medical student; any work undertaken by the student remains the property of the student subject to locally agreed arrangements discussed in advance with student representatives	Your work should not be passed off as somebody else's Expect clear acknowledgement of the ownership of your work
Provide students with the opportunity to provide the medical school or university with feedback on the usefulness, significance and effectiveness of all aspects of the course, including teaching	You may be asked to comment on teaching, support, assessment, organisation and communication
Give due consideration to feedback provided by medical students and inform students of the action that will be taken in response to the feedback	If changes cannot be made in response to your feedback, you should be informed of this
Inform the student, within a reasonable time period, of any changes to the curriculum, structure of the course and any other significant changes other than minor timetabling changes which will affect the student	Ideally, you should be informed of substantial changes one year before they occur (or as soon as possible); such changes include a change of clinical attachment teaching, major course changes, change of university or clinical venue (anything that will require significant expenditure or inconvenience on the student's behalf)
Ensure that medical students have adequate access to modern information technology (IT) equipment that is appropriate to the demands of the course	You will be expected to word-process your reports, therefore you can expect access to appropriate facilities All medical schools should strive to achieve 24-hour access to IT facilities; however, not all have managed this to date

(continued)

Standard: your medical school should . . .	Further details of the standards that should be met by the medical school
Ensure that the student has access to high-quality facilities and resources required to achieve the academic and professional goals set by the GMC and the school	You are required to have a clear understanding of a number of key science subjects, therefore you should have access to anatomical models, professional computer programs, overhead projectors and other resources to achieve this You should not be required to purchase the required items
Ensure all staff with responsibilities to medical students are made aware of the Medical School Charter	The Medical School Charter should be advertised to staff and students
All parties should aim to meet the standards contained in the Medical School Charter	–
Facilitate a high standard of teaching facilities whilst on placement	–
Ensure adequate resources are made available to deliver the relevant parts of the Medical School Charter	–

Standards medical schools are expected to meet regarding accommodation during clinical placements

Council of Heads of Medical Schools and British Medical Association Medical Students Committee. *Medical Student Charter, 2005*. (Available at: www.bma.org. uk/ap.nsf/Content/MedSchCharter)

Standard: your medical school must . . .	Further details of the standards that should be met by the medical school
Provide free accommodation whilst the student is on a placement that is a significant distance from term-time residence	Your medical school should endeavour to supply free accommodation when a clinical attachment is more than one hour from the medical school campus
Ensure that any accommodation provided for students meets HIMOR standards	HIMOR = Housing (Management of Houses in Multiple Occupation) Regulations, 1990 (*see* www. opsi.gov.uk/si/si1990/Uksi_19900830_en_1.htm)

Standards medical schools are expected to meet regarding privacy, equal opportunity, support and student representation

Council of Heads of Medical Schools and British Medical Association Medical Students Committee. *Medical Student Charter, 2005*. (Available at: www.bma.org. uk/ap.nsf/Content/MedSchCharter)

Standard: your medical school must . . .	Further details of the standards that should be met by the medical school
Respect the fundamental human rights of students, as set out by the Human Rights Act 1998 (see www.opsi.gov.uk/ACTS/ acts1998/19980042.htm)	Fundamental human rights include lifestyle, culture, religion and beliefs, race, colour, gender, sexuality, disability, age, nationality or social or economic status
Ensure that learning, both at the medical school and on clinical placements, is undertaken in a safe and secure physical environment	Medical schools must maintain strict health and safety regulations
Provide a diverse environment which takes positive action to protect students from bullying, discrimination, victimisation, intimidation or harassment of any kind, and promotes equality and values diversity	Students and staff must be treated respectfully and not be subject to any form of discrimination. If you report bullying, discrimination, victimisation, intimidation or harassment it should be followed up. Staff members found not to follow up such reports should be excluded from teaching medical students subject to the correct procedures being followed
Provides the student with confidential information and advice on how to make a complaint and whistle-blowing procedures; these complaints shall remain confidential at all times and the complainant shall be protected from any form of victimisation following such a complaint (whether or not such a complaint is upheld)	Clear policies should be available to you to help you and your medical school to take the issue seriously. Treatment of a complaint, whether against staff or student, should be treated in a uniform manner and confidentially

(continued)

Standard: your medical school must . . .	Further details of the standards that should be met by the medical school
Provide access to a student-centred support service within the medical school and ensure that contact with the support service shall be treated in confidence	Your medical school should be able to direct you to facilities within the school that will offer you appropriate and suitable support
Ensure the student has access to both identifiable academic tutors responsible for overseeing education, and identifiable pastoral tutors, to oversee general welfare and assist with personal problems	Your academic and pastoral welfare must be catered for. If a 'conflict of interest' is likely, you should be given information about, and access to, alternative services
Ensure that the role of pastoral tutor does not conflict so as to negatively impact upon the academic progression of the student	Ideally, your pastoral tutor should not also have academic responsibility for you
Ensure that issues disclosed to the pastoral tutor remain confidential; the tutor must advise the student that, in some circumstances, they will be required to disclose information which affects the student's fitness to practice	The student–tutor relationship reflects patient–doctor relationships unless the issue being discussed affects/potentially affects fitness to practice
The medical school should make arrangements for the provision of external support services should these be necessary; it should ensure that the student is aware of these external support mechanisms (including those available through local government and health service providers)	This is particularly relevant for 'embarrassing' issues such as genitourinary and psychiatric problems. Your medical school may have a reciprocal arrangement with other schools. Your medical school should advertise external facilities in case they are required
Ensure that the university provides advice about internal and external sources of funding, including access to hardship funds	–
Ensure that all students have easy access to medical school regulations and policy	–
Ensure that appropriate careers advice is given to students throughout the degree	You should be given advice at suitable times throughout the course If you decide not to pursue a medical career, your medical school should ensure you have access to appropriate career advice
Ensure that, in conjunction with the postgraduate dean, the transition between medical school and F1 year is as seamless as possible; this includes providing information about the process for applying to F1 and how decisions are made	You can expect the application process to be equitable, open, transparent and clearly available To facilitate your application, you should expect suitable career advice
Ensure that the students can make a complaint if they feel they have been treated incorrectly and that any complaint procedure adapted by the medical school is open, transparent and fair as understood by the Human Rights Act	You should have the opportunity, if required, to make an anonymous report of incidents without fear of comeback

(continued)

Standard: your medical school must . . .	Further details of the standards that should be met by the medical school
Ensure that students have access to an internal appeals mechanism and an external appeals panel	It is strongly recommended that an independent student and/or representative of the student body be closely involved in internal appeal processes
Ensure that fair student representation exists on all decision-making bodies which directly affect medical students	All internal bodies that have an effect on medical students should have representation from at least one member of the medical student body; it is strongly recommended that this be extended to representation on appeal bodies and any clinical/academic group
Facilitate the ability of students to participate in all activities of the medical school students' union and external bodies related to education, including trades unions and professional bodies	Representation is a key right. Fair representation should be actively pursued on all key bodies within the medical school. Medical schools should respect a student's right to sit on external bodies in a national or local representative role

References

Notes to Chapter 1: Introduction

1 Royal College of Physicians. *Doctors in Society: medical professionalism in a changing world*. Report of a Working Party of the Royal College of Physicians of London. London: Royal College of Physicians; 2005.

2 Health Policy and Economic Research Unit. *Medical Students Welfare Survey: report*. London: British Medical Association; 2006.

3 British Medical Association Medical Students Committee. *Medicine in the 21st Century: standards for the delivery of undergraduate medical education*. London: British Medical Association; 2005.

4 Council of Heads of Medical Schools and British Medical Association Medical Students Committee. Medical Student Charter. 2005. (Available at: www.bma. org.uk/ap.nsf/Content/MedSchCharter)

Notes to Chapter 2: Medical school: the early days

1 National Union of Students. *Students and Crime: the facts*. (Available at: www. nusonline.co.uk/info/crimeprevention/13269.aspx)

2 Anatomy learning hampered by donated body shortage. *Student BMA News*. 2006; **May**: 3.

3 Morgan J. Do tomorrow's doctors really know no anatomy? *StudentBMJ*. 2006; **14**: 246–7.

4 Available at: http://en.wikipedia.org/wiki/Alcoholic_beverages_%E2%80%94 _recommended_maximum_intake

Note to Chapter 3: People you will meet

1 Porter R. *Blood and Guts: a short history of medicine*. London: Allen Lane; 2002.

Notes to Chapter 4: Competitiveness

1 Winston R. *Human Instinct: how our primeval impulses shape our modern lives*. London: Bantam Press; 2002.

2 Dawkins R. *The Selfish Gene*. 2nd ed. Oxford: Oxford University Press; 1989.

Notes to Chapter 5: Attitude and behaviour

1 Spencer J. Decline in empathy in medical education: how can we stop the rot? *Med Ed.* 2004; **38**: 916–20.

2 General Medical Council. *Tomorrow's Doctors*. London: General Medical Council; 1993.

3 Council of Heads of Medical Schools and British Medical Association Medical Students Committee. Medical Student Charter. 2005. (Available at: www.bma. org.uk/ap.nsf/Content/MedSchCharter)

4 Hebert K. Attitudes decline in medical school. *StudentBMJ.* 2004; **12**: 227.

5 General Medical Council. *The Duties of a Doctor Registered with the General Medical Council*. (Available from: www.gmc-uk.org/standards/doad.htm)

6 Royal College of Physicians. *Doctors in Society: medical professionalism in a changing world*. Report of a Working Party of the Royal College of Physicians of London. London: RCP; 2005.

7 Hilton SR, Slotnick HB. Proto-professionalism: how professionalism occurs across the continuum of medical education. *Med Ed.* 2005; **39**: 58–65.

8 General Medical Council. *Good Medical Practice*. London: General Medical Council; 2006. (Available at: www.gmc-uk.org/med-ed/default.htm)

9 Papadakis MA, Hodgson CS, Teherani A, Kohatsu ND. Unprofessional behaviour in medical school is associated with subsequent disciplinary action by a state medical board. *Acad Med.* 2004; **79**: 244–9.

10 Smith R. Thoughts for new medical students at a new medical school. *BMJ.* 2003; **327**: 1430–3.

11 Glick SM. Cheating at medical school. *BMJ.* 2001; **322**: 250–1.

12 McGinn K. It's all about attitude. *StudentBMJ.* 2006; **14**: 130.

13 Rosenfield PJ, Jones L. Striking a balance: training medical students to provide empathetic care. *Med Ed.* 2004; **38**: 927–33.

Notes to Chapter 6: Course structure

1 General Medical Council. *Tomorrow's Doctors: recommendations on undergraduate medical education*. London: General Medical Council; 2003.

2 General Medical Council. *Good Medical Practice*. London: General Medical Council; 2006. (Available at: www.gmc-uk.org/med-ed/default.htm)

3 Wass V. Ensuring medical students are 'fit for purpose'. *BMJ.* 2005; **331**: 791–2.

4 Rubin P. *Core Education Outcomes: GMC Education Committee position statement*. London: General Medical Council; 2006.

5 McManus IC, Richards P, Winder BC. Intercalated degrees, learning styles and career preferences: prospective longitudinal study of UK medical students. *BMJ.* 1999; **319**: 542–6.

6 Wood DF. ABC of learning and teaching in medicine: problem based learning. *BMJ.* 2003; **326**: 328–30.

7 Leung WC. Is PBL better than traditional curriculum? *StudentBMJ*. 2001; **9**: 306–7.

8 Morgan J. Do tomorrow's doctors really know no anatomy? *StudentBMJ*. 2006; **14**: 246–7.

9 Tiwari A, Lai P, So M, Yuen K. A comparison of the effects of problem-based learning and lecturing on the development of students' critical thinking. *Med Ed*. 2006; **40**: 547–54.

10 Kassem A. Students and teachers prefer early experience. *StudentBMJ*. 2004; **12**: 396.

11 Goelen G, De Clercq G, Huyghens L, Kerchofs E. Measuring the effect of interprofessional problem-based learning on the attitudes of undergraduate health care students. *Med Ed*. 2006; **40**: 555–61.

Notes to Chapter 7: Learning

1 Powell M. *The Little Book of Crap Advice*. London: Michael O'Mara Books; 2001.

2 Council of Heads of Medical Schools and British Medical Association Medical Students Committee. Medical Student Charter. 2005. (Available at: www.bma. org.uk/ap.nsf/Content/MedSchCharter)

3 Spencer JA, Jordan RK. Learner centred approaches in medical education. *BMJ*. 1999; **318**: 1280–3.

4 Baddeley A. *Human Memory: theory and practice*. Revised ed. London: Psychology Press Ltd; 1999.

5 General Medical Council. *Tomorrow's Doctors: recommendations on undergraduate medical education*. London: General Medical Council; 2003.

6 McManus IC, Richards P, Winder PC, Sproston KA. Clinical experience, performance in final examinations, and learning style in medical students: prospective study. *BMJ*. 1998; **316**: 345–50.

7 Longmore M, Wilkinson I, Török E. *Oxford Handbook of Clinical Medicine*. Fifth ed. Oxford: Oxford University Press; 2001.

8 Jenkins D, Gerred S. *ECGs by Example*. Edinburgh: Churchill Livingstone; 1997.

9 http://en.wikipedia.org/wiki/William_Osler

Notes to Chapter 8: Exams

1 General Medical Council. *Tomorrow's Doctors: recommendations on undergraduate medical education*. London: GMC; 2003.

2 Cantillon P. Mastering exam technique. *StudentBMJ*. 2000; **8**: 363–5.

3 Chen S. How to answer MCQs. *StudentBMJ*. 2005; **13**: 110.

4 Bickle I. Mastering EMQs. *StudentBMJ*. 2002; **10**: 406–7.

5 Clarke R. How to Approach Clinical Examinations in Medicine. (Available at: www.askdoctorclarke.com)

6 Wass V. Getting through OSCEs. *StudentBMJ*. 2000; **8**: 361–2.

7 Setchell M, Thilaganathan B. *Ten Teachers' Self Assessment in Gynaecology and Obstetrics*. 4th ed. London: Arnold; 2001.

8 Smith G, Carty E, Langmead L. *Pass Finals: a companion to Kumar and Clark*. Edinburgh: Churchill Livingstone; 2004.

9 Lissauer T, Roberts G, Foster C, Coren M. *Illustrated Self Assessment in Paediatrics*. Edinburgh: Elsevier; 2001.

10 Baliga RR. *MCQs in Clinical Medicine*. 2nd ed. Edinburgh: WB Saunders; 2003.

11 Wass V. Ensuring medical students are 'fit for purpose'. *BMJ*. 2005; **331**: 791–2.

Notes to Chapter 9: Projects

1 Royal College of Physicians. *Doctors in Society: medical professionalism in a changing world*. Report of a Working Party of the Royal College of Physicians of London. London: Royal College of Physicians; 2005.

2 Sackett DL, Rosenberg WMC, Gray JAM, Haynes RB, Richardson WS. Evidence-based medicine: what it is and what it isn't. *BMJ*. 1996; **312**: 71–2.

3 Greenhalgh T. *How to Read a Paper: the basics of evidence based medicine*. London: BMJ Publishing Group; 2000.

4 Calvache JA. Evidence based medicine. *StudentBMJ*. 2006; **14**: 307.

5 Sackett DL, Straus SE, Richardson WS, Rosenberg W, Haynes RB. *Evidence-based Medicine: how to practice and teach EBM*. 3rd ed. Edinburgh: Churchill Livingstone; 2005.

6 Scally G, Donaldson LJ. Clinical governance and the drive for quality improvement in the new NHS in England. *BMJ*. 1998; **317**: 61–5.

7 South Stoke Teaching Primary Care Trust. *Clinical Governance Handbook*. Stoke on Trent: National Health Service; 2003.

8 Cates C. *Understanding Statistics 2: is there a significant difference?* (Interactive case history); 2006. (Available at: www.bmjlearning.com)

9 Linda Thompson (performs), Denny S. *I'm a Dreamer. Dreams Fly Away: a history of Linda Thompson*. Hannibal; 1996.

Notes to Chapter 10: Oral presentations

1 Diver AJ. Tips on presenting to a clinical audience. *StudentBMJ*. 2005; **13**: 377.

2 Raveenthiran V. The 10 commandments of oral presentations. *StudentBMJ*. 2005; **13**: 374–5.

3 Natarajan A, Kirby JA. A guide to oral presentation skills. *StudentBMJ*. 2005; **13**: 376–7.

Notes to Chapter 11: Let's talk money

1 British Medical Association. *Medicine in the 21st Century: standards for the delivery of undergraduate medical education*. London: BMA; 2005.

2 British Medical Association. *The Survey of Medical Students' Finances 2004–5*. London: British Medical Association; 2005.

3 www.bma.org.uk/ap.nsf/Content/Hubstudentbmanews

4 British Medical Association. Graduation debt: survey reveals £20,000 average. *StudentBMA News*. 2006; **Jan**: 3.

5 www.money4medicalstudents.org

6 www.aimhigher.ac.uk

7 South Central Connexions. *Let's Talk About Higher Education at 18+*. Hampshire: Connexions; 2006.

8 Independent Committee of Inquiry into Student Finances. *Student Finance: fairness for the future*. Scotland: Scottish Executive; 1999.

9 www.bl.uk/collections/social/welfare/issue10/eduhigh.html

Notes to Chapter 12: *Life away from medicine*

1 Council of Heads of Medical Schools and British Medical Association Medical Students Committee. Medical Student Charter. 2005. (Available at: www.bma.org.uk/ap.nsf/Content/MedSchCharter)

2 Delia Smith. *Complete Illustrated Cookery Course*. Classic edition. London: BBC Books; 2000.

3 Sladden J. Medical marriages. *StudentBMJ*. 2004; **12**: 472–3.

4 Health Policy and Economic Research Unit. *Medical Students Welfare Survey: report*. London: British Medical Association; 2006.

5 British Medical Association Medical Students Committee. *Medical Student Welfare Survey*. London: British Medical Association; 2004.

Notes to Chapter 14: *When things go wrong*

1 Powell M. *The Little Book of Crap Advice*. London: Michael O'Mara Books; 2001.

2 Adams T. Medical school culture: exam failure. *StudentBMJ*. 2001; **9**: 484.

3 General Medical Council. *Tomorrow's Doctors: recommendations on undergraduate medical education*. London: General Medical Council; 2003.

4 British Medical Association Medical Students Committee. *Medicine in the 21st Century: standards for the delivery of undergraduate medical education*. London: British Medical Association; 2005.

5 Health Policy and Economic Research Unit. *Medical Students Welfare Survey: report*. London: British Medical Association; 2006.

6 Council of Heads of Medical Schools and British Medical Association Medical Students Committee. Medical Student Charter. 2005. (Available at: www.bma.org.uk/ap.nsf/Content/MedSchCharter)

7 Oxley J. *Supporting Doctors and Nurses at Work: an enquiry into mentoring*. London: SCOPME; 1998.

8 British Medical Association Board of Medical Education. *Exploring Mentoring*. London: British Medical Association; 2004.

9 Robinson G, Bernau S, Aldington S, Beasley R. From medical student to junior doctor: maintaining good health during the 'baptism of fire'. *StudentBMJ*. 2006; **14**: 138–9.

10 Locke M. Are you fit to practise. *StudentBMJ*. 2006; **14**: 68–9.

11 Royal College of Psychiatrists. *The Mental Health of Students in Higher Education*. London: Royal College of Psychiatrists; 2003.

12 Minck S. *Managing Stress*. (Available at: <u>www.doctors.net.uk/targetting/Article.</u> <u>aspx?articleid=874&areaid=11</u>)

13 Murdoch-Eaton D. Student appraisal: a model for the future. *The Clinical Teacher*. 2006; **3**: 138–42.

14 Gangwisch JE, Heymsfield SB, Boden-Albala B *et al.* Short sleep duration as a risk factor for hypertension: analysis of the first National Health and Nutrition Examination Survey. *Hypertension*. 2006; **47**: 833–9.

15 MacDonald R. Eating disorders: medical students with 'disordered eating' need to be supported not judged. *StudentBMJ*. 2001; **9**: 219–21.

16 Szweda S, Thorne P. The prevalence of eating disorders in female health care students. *Occup Med*. 2002; **52**: 113–19.

17 Medical Council on Alcohol. (Available at: <u>www.medicouncilalcol.demon.</u> <u>co.uk/prac_alc.htm</u>)

Note to Chapter 15: How to get the most from medical school

1 General Medical Council. *Tomorrow's Doctors: recommendations on undergraduate medical education*. London: General Medical Council; 2003. (Available at: <u>www.</u> <u>gmc-uk.org</u>)

Note to Appendix III: Standards medical schools are expected to meet regarding education, training and facilities

1 General Medical Council. *Tomorrow's Doctors: recommendations on undergraduate medical education*. London: General Medical Council; 2003.

Index